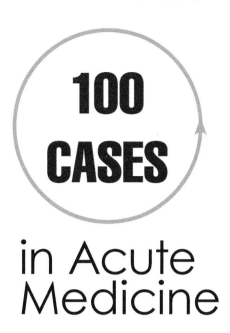

100 CASES

in Acute Medicine

100 Cases in Acute Medicine presents 100 acute conditions commonly seen by medical students and junior doctors in the emergency department or on the ward or in the community setting. A succinct summary of the patient's history, examination and initial investigations, including photographs where relevant, is followed by questions on the diagnosis and management of each case. The answer includes a detailed discussion on each topic, with further illustration where appropriate, providing an essential revision aid, as well as a practical guide for students and junior doctors.

Making clinical decisions and choosing the best course of action is one of the most challenging and difficult parts of training to become a doctor. Fully revised and updated for this second edition, these cases will teach students and junior doctors to recognise important clinical symptoms and signs and to develop their diagnostic and management skills.

About the Series

Making speedy and appropriate clinical decisions, and choosing the best course of action to take as a result, is one of the most important and challenging parts of training to become a doctor. The real-life cases presented in the 100 Cases series encompass emergency, ward, and outpatient and community scenarios, and have been designed specifically to help medical students and junior doctors to develop their diagnostic and management skills.

100 Diagnostic Dilemmas in Clinical Medicine
Kerry Layne

100 Cases in General Practice, 2E
Anne E. Stephenson, Martin Mueller, John Grabinar

100 Cases in Clinical Pharmacology, Therapeutics and Prescribing
Kerry Layne, Albert Ferro

100 Cases in Acute Medicine
Henry Fok, Kerry Layne and Adam Nabeebaccus

For more information about this series please visit: www.routledge.com/100-Cases/book-series/CRCONEHUNCAS

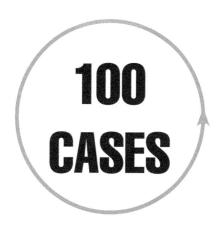

100 CASES

in Acute Medicine
Second Edition

Henry Fok
Honorary Consultant Physician,
St George's University Hospitals NHS Foundation Trust,
London, UK

Kerry Layne
Consultant in Acute Medicine,
Guy's & St Thomas' NHS Foundation Trust,
London, UK

Adam Nabeebaccus
Honorary Consultant in Cardiology,
King's College Hospital NHS Foundation Trust,
London, UK

100 Cases Series Editor:
Janice Rymer MBBS, FRACP
Professor of Obstetrics & Gynaecology and
Dean of Student Affairs, King's College London
School of Medicine, London, UK

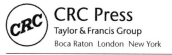

CRC Press
Taylor & Francis Group
Boca Raton London New York

CRC Press is an imprint of the
Taylor & Francis Group, an **informa** business

Second edition published 2023
by CRC Press
6000 Broken Sound Parkway NW, Suite 300, Boca Raton, FL 33487–2742

and by CRC Press
4 Park Square, Milton Park, Abingdon, Oxon, OX14 4RN

CRC Press is an imprint of Taylor & Francis Group, LLC

© 2023 Henry Fok, Kerry Layne and Adam Nabeebaccus

First edition published by CRC Press 2012

Library of Congress Cataloging-in-Publication Data
[Insert LoC Data here when available]

ISBN: 978-1-032-14803-8 (hbk)
ISBN: 978-1-032-14801-4 (pbk)
ISBN: 978-1-003-24117-1 (ebk)

DOI: 10.1201/9781003241171

Typeset in Baskerville
by Apex CoVantage, LLC

CONTENTS

ABBREVIATIONS

ABG   arterial blood gas
ALP   alkaline phosphatase
ALT   alanine aminotransferase
BE   Base excess
Bili   bilirubin
BP   blood pressure
BD   twice daily
Creat creatinine
CRP   C-reactive protein
CT   computed tomography
DKA   diabetic ketoacidosis
ECG   electrocardiogram
EEG   electroencephalogram
GTN   glyceryl trinitrate
Hb   haemoglobin
HbA1c glycated haemoglobin
HIV   human immunodeficiency virus
HR   heart rate
JVP   jugular venous pressure
K   potassium
LMWH   low molecular weight heparin
MRI   magnetic resonance imaging
Na   sodium
NIV   non-invasive ventilation
OD   once daily
Plt   platelet count
QDS   four times daily
RNA   ribonucleic acid
RR   respiratory rate
SBP   systolic blood pressure
SpO2   peripheral capillary oxygen saturations
TDS   three times daily
VBG   venous blood gas
WCC   white cell count

CASE 1: ACUTE CONFUSION

History

A 65-year-old woman is found wandering the streets in a confused and agitated state, so passers-by call for an ambulance. The patient is unable to give a thorough history. Her neighbours inform the paramedics that she is usually fit and well, although her past medical history is significant for bipolar affective disorder, for which she takes lithium. Her other regular medications are ramipril and bendroflumethiazide for hypertension. She lives alone and attends a drop-in community mental health centre in addition to regular visits by a community psychiatric nurse and a friend. She denies smoking or drinking alcohol.

Examination

Observations: temperature 37.4°C, heart rate 42/min, blood pressure 128/84 mmHg, respiratory rate 20/min, SpO$_2$ 99% on room air. No injuries are visible. Her mucous membranes appear dry. Cardiovascular, respiratory, and abdominal examinations are unremarkable. Neurological examination identifies a coarse, irregular tremor in all four limbs, as well as symmetrically increased tone in the lower limbs, and an extrapyramidal gait.

🔍 INVESTIGATIONS

- Her lithium level is 3 mmol/L (therapeutic reference interval 0.4–1.0 mmol/L).
- An ECG is shown in Figure 1.1.

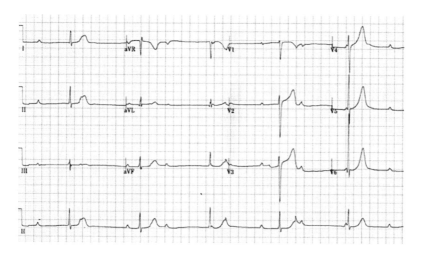

Figure 1.1

❓ QUESTIONS

1. What is the most likely diagnosis?
2. What signs and symptoms should you be cautious of?
3. What does the ECG show?
4. How will you manage this patient acutely?

DOI: 10.1201/9781003241171-1

ANSWERS

The patient is on lithium, so toxicity should always be suspected. Lithium has a narrow therapeutic window, and toxicity can occur at levels greater than 1.4 mmol/L. Patients are particularly prone to developing lithium toxicity when they are dehydrated (e.g. secondary to diarrhoea and vomiting) or if they have renal impairment. Use of sodium-depleting drugs, such as thiazide diuretics and angiotensin-converting enzyme inhibitors, can also predispose a person to lithium toxicity.

Symptoms of lithium toxicity usually begin with gastrointestinal disturbances, such as nausea, vomiting, and diarrhoea. This can then progress to neurological symptoms, such as ataxia and confusion. Neurological examination may identify hyperreflexia, hypertonia, and nystagmus. Seizures may develop and eventually progress to coma. Increased resistance to the antidiuretic hormone (ADH) can occur in lithium toxicity, resulting in the development of nephrogenic diabetes insipidus and subsequent chronic kidney disease. Patients on lithium should have regular monitoring of their renal function in order to detect this at an early, and potentially reversible, stage.

The ECG shows third-degree atrioventricular block, also known as complete heart block. The P waves show a regular P-P interval. The QRS complexes also demonstrate a regular R-R interval. The P-R interval is variable, and there appears to be no relationship between the P waves and the QRS complexes. This is because the impulses generated by the sinoatrial node do not propagate down to the ventricles, and the rhythms of the atria and the ventricles are completely dissociated. Because the sinoatrial node cannot conduct to the ventricles, an accessory pacemaker site farther down the cardiac tissue can develop and activate the ventricles, leading to an escape rhythm.

Lithium toxicity can also lead to cardiotoxicity. First-degree heart block, where the duration of the P-R interval is increased, commonly develops. This can progress to complete heart block, as in this case. Patients with complete heart block are at high risk of hypotensive, bradycardic episodes and life-threatening arrhythmias. This woman should be placed on a cardiac monitor to observe her cardiac rhythm, and she may need a temporary pacing wire to be sited. Fortunately, in this case, the heart block resolved without any intervention being required.

Your focus should be to prevent seizures and the development of renal failure or cardiotoxicity. Lithium is completely absorbed by the gastrointestinal tract and then renally excreted. Owing to the complete heart block, the patient is at risk of further abnormal rhythms, including asystole.

Those with mild lithium toxicity (1.5–2.5 mmol/L) who appear clinically well and are asymptomatic should be monitored closely. You must ensure they are passing good volumes of urine. Increased oral intake of fluid and intravenous fluids may be necessary.

People with lithium levels >2.5 mmol/L typically need to be admitted to hospital for in-patient management. The patient should be placed on a cardiac monitor, and senior medical staff should be involved early.

If the overdose was taken within the last few hours, advice should be sought from a poisons centre as to whether methods such as gastric lavage or whole-bowel irrigation are recommended. Activated charcoal ingestion offers no benefit with lithium, as the ions do not bind to the charcoal. Intravenous fluid therapy should be commenced early, and haemodialysis can be considered to remove the lithium from the circulation. Drugs to alkalinise the urine may help improve lithium excretion.

Lithium levels in the blood will need to be monitored frequently. If the patient is not improving, their care should be escalated to a critical care setting.

🔑 **KEY POINTS**

1. Monitor lithium levels in patients using this drug. Lithium toxicity can be very dangerous, leading to multi-organ failure.
2. When a person presents with lithium toxicity, involve senior doctors early.
3. Perform blood tests to check renal function, and ensure the patient stays on a cardiac monitor if they have ECG abnormalities or signs of cardiac dysfunction.
4. Haemodialysis may be required to remove lithium from the body.

CASE 2: APPARENT ADVERSE DRUG REACTION

History

A 64-year-old woman is admitted to hospital with shortness of breath and a cough productive of dark green sputum. She is treated in the emergency department with intravenous fluid rehydration and intravenous amoxicillin with clavulanic acid for presumed community-acquired pneumonia. Her past medical history includes osteoarthritis of the left knee and depression. She takes no regular medications and has no known allergies. Five minutes after administration of the antibiotic, she complains of feeling short of breath and light-headed.

Examination

The patient looks very pale and appears short of breath. There is an erythematous, macular rash over her cheeks and on her trunk. The patient is unable to speak in full sentences due to dyspnoea. Her temperature is 37.5°C. She is tachycardic with a heart rate of 130 beats per minute and hypotensive with a blood pressure of 80/42 mmHg. On auscultation of her chest, there is an audible wheeze; her respiratory rate is 24 breaths per minute, and her peripheral oxygen saturations are 96% on room air.

? QUESTIONS

1. What is the most likely diagnosis?
2. How would you manage this patient acutely?
3. Once she is clinically stable, what management plan would you suggest?

DOI: 10.1201/9781003241171-2

ANSWERS

1. This woman is likely having an anaphylactic reaction to the penicillin-based anti-biotic. Anaphylaxis is a systemic reaction to an allergen, leading to degranulation of mast cells and basophils and the release of histamine and other inflammatory mediators. Initial clinical features can include a rash, facial swelling, hypotension, tachycardia, and wheeze. Patients may subsequently develop laryngeal oedema, bronchospasm, and circulatory collapse. This is a life-threatening condition and needs to be recognised and treated urgently.

2. The acute management of anaphylaxis can be lifesaving and should be commenced as soon as you suspect the diagnosis. The first step is to remove the allergen, for example, by stopping the intravenous infusion of antibiotics and, ideally, removing the intravenous cannula through which it was administered so that any residual anti-biotic does not enter the circulation when the cannula is next used (if further venous access cannot be rapidly obtained, then it may be considered safer to keep the can-nula in situ). In a hospital-based setting, there should be an anaphylaxis kit on every ward, which is usually placed on the crash trolley in a yellow box. You should ensure that senior help is available, either by putting out a crash call in a hospital or calling emergency services if in the community.

If the patient has signs of respiratory or cardiovascular compromise, immediately administer 0.5 mg adrenaline intramuscularly (0.5 mL, 1:1000). Adrenaline will act rapidly, within seconds to minutes, with α-adrenergic effects (vasoconstriction) and β-adrenergic effects (bronchial dilation).

Manage the Patient Using the ABC Pathway

A: Airway—assess that the airway is patent. Call for anaesthetic support if the airway is compromised and use basic life support techniques (head tilt, chin lift, jaw thrust).

B: Breathing—auscultate the praecordium and observe the chest wall movement to ensure equal and symmetrical movement. Monitor the respiratory rate and the oxygen saturations. In the acute setting, apply 15 L oxygen via a non-rebreather mask if the patient is dyspnoeic or desaturating. If you can hear wheeze, admin-ister a bronchodilator, such as a salbutamol nebuliser followed by a muscarinic agonist, such as an ipratropium bromide nebuliser. Consider doing an arterial blood gas test to assess for hypoxia or hypercapnia.

C: Circulation—monitor the heart rate and blood pressure. Tachycardia and hypo-tension are signs of circulatory compromise. Listen to the patient's heart; check the pulse and the capillary refill time. Ensure the patient has intravenous access with a large-bore cannula. Start intravenous fluids, and increase the rate of flow if the patient is hypotensive.

Remember that although adrenaline acts rapidly, it also has a short duration of action; consider giving another dose if necessary. Alongside adrenaline, you should also administer 200 mg hydrocortisone intramuscularly or intravenously. This is a corticosteroid that acts to decrease eosinophil action and generally reduce the inflammatory response. Remember that corticosteroids typically take sev-eral hours to have a significant effect. Next, administer 10 mg chlorpheniramine intramuscularly or intravenously. Chlorpheniramine is a histamine H_1 receptor agonist and can prevent the excess histamine generated in response to an allergen from triggering further immune responses, but it also takes over an hour to exert any significant effect.

3. The patient will need to be reviewed by a senior doctor and should be monitored closely for a further 24 hours. Around one in five patients develops a late-phase ana-phylactic reaction 4–8 hours after the initial episode, despite no further exposure to the allergen. This occurs when neutrophils and eosinophils migrate to the site of the initial allergen recognition and generate a further inflammatory response. Additionally, cytokines released from mast cells may remain present for several hours, provoking ongoing inflammation.

Intravenous fluid rehydration should be continued for 4–6 hours, and the patient will need regular monitoring to review whether they need further doses of adren-aline and nebulisers. The patient should be informed that they have had a life-threatening allergic response to a penicillin-based drug and that they should inform medical staff of this whenever they attend hospital or are prescribed medications in the community. Her medical records must be updated to reflect this allergy, and her general practitioner will need to be informed. An allergy bracelet should be worn during her hospital stay and for any future admissions. If there is doubt about the precipitant of the anaphylactic reaction, an allergy clinic referral should be made where allergy testing can be performed in a safe environment.

🔑 KEY POINTS

1. Always ask a patient if they have any known allergies when taking a history. This includes food allergies.
2. Anaphylaxis is a medical emergency. Treat patients immediately with intramuscular adrenaline and call for help as soon as possible.
3. Manage patients according to the ABC principles. Are your basic life support skills up to date?
4. Remember that some combination antibiotics, such as Augmentin (co-amoxiclav) and Tazocin (piperacillin/tazobactam) are penicillin-based, so always check whether an antibiotic contains a penicillin before prescribing it.

CASE 3: SHORTNESS OF BREATH AND A COUGH

History

A 64-year-old Afro-Caribbean woman presents to the emergency department complaining of shortness of breath. She has been feeling generally unwell for several weeks and has become increasingly breathless over the past 4 days. She describes a non-productive cough but denies any fevers or night sweats. Her medical history is significant for a recent diagnosis of right-sided carcinoma of the breast that was treated with a lumpectomy (removal of the tumour in the breast) and a course of chemotherapy.

Examination

The patient looks comfortably at rest but becomes short of breath on minimal exertion. She is afebrile. There are reduced breath sounds on the right side of her chest, with right-sided dullness to percussion. Her oxygen saturations are 90% on room air. A chest x-ray is performed in the emergency department (Figure 3.1).

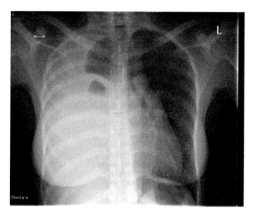

Figure 3.1

? QUESTIONS

1. What does the chest x-ray show?
2. How would you investigate the underlying cause?
3. What would be the best treatment to help this patient's symptoms?

DOI: 10.1201/9781003241171-3

ANSWERS

1. The chest x-ray shows a large, right-sided pleural effusion, as indicated by the opacification of the right lung fields and loss of the costophrenic angle. This is often called a "white-out" appearance. The mediastinum (heart, great vessels, trachea, and oesophagus) has been pushed towards the left side of the chest.

2. A sample of the fluid is needed. Pleural fluid can be aspirated using a needle (thoracocentesis or pleural tap) and then analysed. An ultrasound probe should be used to identify exactly where the effusion is present, and then a needle can be safely inserted, ideally into the "safe triangle" area—a triangle bordered by the mid-axillary line, the lateral border of the pectoralis major muscle, a line superior to the horizontal level of the nipple, and an apex below the axilla.

   The fluid should be inspected grossly: is it blood-stained or straw coloured? Does it appear viscous? These features will all give us clues as to the underlying cause of the effusion. Four main types of fluid accumulate in the pleural space—blood (haemothorax), serous fluid (hydrothorax), chyle (chylothorax), and pus (empyema). It is important to test the pH of pleural fluid, as a pH <7.3 indicates the presence of an empyema.

   Transudates tend to be caused by systemic conditions that alter the balance of pleural fluid production and resorption, such as heart failure, renal failure, and liver failure, whilst exudates are more likely to be caused by local conditions, such as bacterial infection or malignancy. Effusions can be classed as transudates or exudates, based on the following criteria:

	Transudate	Exudate
Appearance of pleural fluid	Clear	Turbid
Protein ratio—pleural fluid:serum	<0.5	≥0.5
LDH ratio—pleural fluid:serum	<0.6	≥0.6
Pleural fluid LDH level	<2/3 upper limit of normal serum LDH level	≥2/3 upper limit of normal serum LDH level
Pleural fluid protein level	≤30 g/L	>30 g/L

3. In this case, where the patient has a history of breast cancer, the fluid in her pleural space could be a malignant effusion, which is typically an exudate. It may be that her breast cancer has spread, so further tests will need to be done to identify whether this is the case. With smaller effusions, a thoracocentesis may remove enough fluid to improve symptoms, but in this situation, where there is a large volume of fluid, a chest drain should be inserted.

   Pleural effusions can recur, particularly malignant ones. Patients who develop malignant effusions despite optimal treatment of the malignancy may be referred for a pleurodesis. This involves inducing scarring of the pleura, either chemically or surgically, so that they adhere together to prevent fluid re-accumulating.

🔑 **KEY POINTS**

1. Patients with a pleural effusion will typically have reduced breath sounds and dullness to percussion with decreased vocal resonance and tactile fremitus on the affected side.
2. Pleural fluid can be sampled via thoracocentesis, but a chest drain may be needed for large effusions.
3. Patients who develop malignant effusions may be referred for a pleurodesis.

CASE 4: COLLAPSE AND CONFUSION IN A YOUNG WOMAN

History

A 32-year-old woman collapses while exercising at a gym. Her friends describe the woman falling to the floor, followed by twitching of her arms and legs and then a period of being unrousable. The woman reportedly remembered nothing following her arrival at the gym and was confused and drowsy for 10 minutes following the event. She had bitten her tongue but did not lose continence. She has no past medical history of note, takes no regular medications, and there is no family history of seizures. She has an extensive travel history, having backpacked around Asia on multiple occasions over the past 5 years, staying in hostels and eating at street food stalls. She describes being 'completely fit and well' prior to the event and had not used any medications, alcohol, or recreational drugs or sustained a head injury.

Examination

The woman is alert and fully orientated, and there are no significant findings on examination, including a full neurological assessment.

 INVESTIGATIONS

- An HIV test is negative.
- A CT head scan initially showed a cystic ring-enhancing lesion. Two days later, an MRI head scan was performed and was reported as showing a 13 × 10 × 10 mm ring-enhancing cystic lesion in the left parietal lobe of a 'dot-in-hole' appearance and surrounding mild oedema (Figure 4.1).

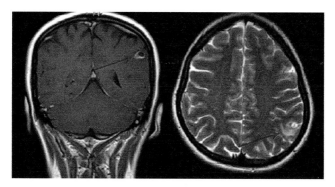

Figure 4.1

? **QUESTION**

1. In view of the history and scans, what is the most likely diagnosis?

DOI: 10.1201/9781003241171-4

ANSWERS

This woman has presented with a generalised seizure. Adult-onset epilepsy is uncommon, and other underlying causes of a first fit should be considered, such as a space-occupying lesion or a cerebral bleed, as well as metabolic disturbances.

The CT head scan shows a lesion in the left parietal lobe with a central focus and ring enhancement. The differential diagnosis of ring-enhancing cerebral lesions in patients who are not immunocompromised typically includes primary or secondary tumours and pyogenic abscesses. In immunocompromised patients, consider also *Toxoplasma* infections, lymphoma, and cerebral tuberculosis. This patient's HIV test was negative, and she had normal blood counts.

The MRI scan shows the lesion in better detail, revealing the classic 'dot-in-hole' appearance that is associated with neurocysticercosis. This is the most common parasitic infection of the central nervous system and the leading cause of adult-onset seizures in the developing world. The infection has a complex cycle and begins with humans ingesting raw or undercooked pork from pigs infected with *Taenia solium*. Humans can subsequently develop tapeworm infections and shed embryonated eggs in their faeces. In areas with poor hygiene facilities or where human waste is used as a fertiliser, these embryonated eggs can be ingested, leading to cysticerci developing in all tissues, particularly in the brain, eyes, and subcutaneous tissue.

This patient should receive anti-helminth medication. Most patients will remain free of seizures once the underlying structural lesions are broken down. This may take some time following anti-helminth medication, and some people will need to remain on anti-epileptic drugs for months to years.

 KEY POINTS

1. Neurocysticercosis is the most common cause of adult-onset seizures in the developing world and should be considered in all atypical first fits.
2. Always take a full social history from a patient, including travel details, as this can provide vital information regarding exposure to environmental and infectious diseases.

History

An 82-year-old woman has noticed increasing difficulty over recent months when trying to walk upstairs. She is due to have a right-sided hip replacement in a few months' time as a result of severe osteoarthritic changes to her hip joint. She manages her hip pain with paracetamol and dihydrocodeine. When walking upstairs to her bedroom one evening, she trips and falls down eight stairs. She sustains a large laceration to the scalp, which is now bleeding profusely. She telephones her daughter, who immediately calls for an ambulance. On arrival to hospital, the patient was alert and orientated and appeared well. Systems examination, including a full neurological assessment, is unremarkable.

The wound is managed by the emergency department team, who achieve haemostasis and glue the laceration. Following this, the patient is keen to go home. She is assessed by the physiotherapy and occupational therapy teams, who feel it would be safer for the patient to be admitted for a few days to allow a temporary microenvironment to be set up in her home to prevent further falls.

The patient mobilises around the ward and is completely independent with self-care but 3 days later, is found to be confused and drowsy in bed.

On Examination

The patient is unresponsive to pain. Her pupils are only sluggishly responsive to light. Her heart rate has fallen from 88 bpm to 40 bpm, and her blood pressure has risen from 110/60 mmHg to 183/75 mmHg. Her respiratory rate increases from 15 bpm to 26 bpm, and her oxygen requirements increase until her saturations are 91% on 15 L oxygen.

🔍 INVESTIGATIONS

- The patient is assessed by the elderly care junior doctor on call, who arranges an urgent CT head scan (Figure 5.1) (shown here with her observation chart; Figure 5.2).

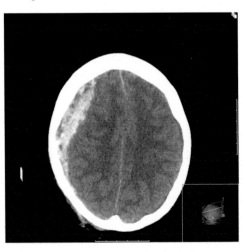

Figure 5.1

DOI: 10.1201/9781003241171-5

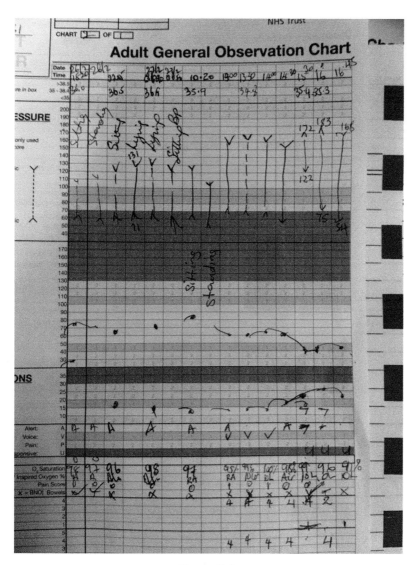

Figure 5.2

? **QUESTIONS**

1. What condition needs to be suspected in this case?
2. What treatment can be given to a patient with these problems?

ANSWERS

1. The main differential diagnosis to consider is a chronic subdural haematoma. Subdural haematomas are bleeds that occur between the dura mater and the arachnoid mater, enveloping the brain. They usually develop following traumatic injury, as with this case. The bridging veins crossing the subdural space tear when head injuries take place, mainly due to the high-speed accelerations and decelerations that occur. Older people are particularly prone to such injuries, as the brain naturally atrophies and shrinks with age. Blood collects in the space and draws in water due to osmotic pressures. The area of bleeding increases in size, causing compression of the cerebral tissue.

   This patient has signs of raised intracranial pressure, as noted by the change in her bedside observations (see chart). Cushing's triad of systolic hypertension with a wide pulse pressure, bradycardia, and irregular or rapid respiratory rate is a major sign of raised intracranial pressure. These features occur due to insufficient blood flow to the brain and compression of arterioles.

   Subacute and chronic subdural haematomas classically present days to weeks after the initial insult. Any patient that presents with new neurological signs several days after a head injury should be investigated for a potential subdural bleed.

2. Ideally, intracranial haemorrhages should be identified as soon as possible to facilitate early treatment. Any patient with a head injury should undergo a neurological examination, and if abnormal signs are present, a CT head scan should be considered, if appropriate. Medical therapies include steroids that can reduce cerebral oedema, medication to reduce bleeding or counteract anticoagulant therapies that the patient may be taking, and anti-epileptic medications to prevent seizures.

   Small bleeds may be monitored over time because if the bleeding has stopped, neurosurgical intervention may not be required. Larger bleeds may require a burr hole to be drilled into the skull to remove a blood clot, or a craniotomy can be performed. Unfortunately, as in this advanced case of a bleed, the haematoma may be inoperable and palliative care will be commenced.

🔑 **KEY POINTS**

1. Always perform a full neurological examination on anyone presenting with a head injury.
2. Have a low threshold for considering a subdural bleed in patients who deteriorate more than 48 hours after their head injury.

CASE 6: CONSTIPATION WITH CONFUSION

History

A 71-year-old man was found to be confused at home, and his daughter brought him to the emergency department to be reviewed. The patient is unable to give any history to the doctors, responding with "yes" to all questions. The patient's daughter reports that he had mentioned becoming increasingly constipated over recent weeks but seemed to be well otherwise. She also said that the patient complained of generalised aches and pains that had been bothering him for a few days, which he had attributed to arthritis, although his general practitioner (GP) had arranged a bone scan to investigate this further. When the patient's daughter visited him earlier in the day, she found him lying in bed, distressed, and with obvious pain in his left arm. He was orientated to person but not time or place.

Examination

The patient appears fairly comfortable at rest, although he is cradling his left arm. On examination his blood pressure was 160/94 mmHg and his pulse was 102 beats per minute.

🔍 INVESTIGATIONS

- An x-ray of his left arm showed a fracture in the mid-shaft of the humerus. He was seen by the orthopaedics team, who felt this was a pathological fracture (Figure 6.1).
- Blood results—WCC 6.0, Hb 11.8, Plt 320, Na 138, K 4.2, creatinine 150, and corrected calcium 3.1.

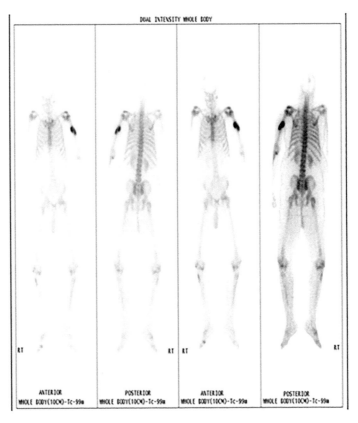

Figure 6.1

DOI: 10.1201/9781003241171-6

- Results from the bone scan and protein electrophoresis are shown in Figure 6.2.

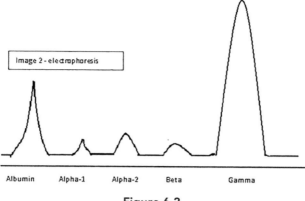

Image 2 - electrophoresis

| Albumin | Alpha-1 | Alpha-2 | Beta | Gamma |

Figure 6.2

? QUESTIONS

1. What is the most probable underlying diagnosis?
2. How could you confirm your suspected diagnosis?
3. What treatment would you give this gentleman in the first 24 hours of his stay?

ANSWERS

1. This gentleman has symptoms of hypercalcaemia ("bones, stones, abdominal groans, and psychic moans") and, based on the results of his investigations, is likely to have multiple myeloma.

   Multiple myeloma is a cancer of the plasma cells in the blood, which are responsible for producing antibodies. These abnormal cells form collections in bony spaces (plasmacytomas) which cause lytic lesions and predispose to pathological fractures (i.e. fractures that are unexpected given the history, with no appropriate traumatic cause).

   Plasmacytomas can also accumulate in the bone marrow, leading to impaired haematopoiesis. Patients present with symptoms related to poor red cell production (pallor, fatigue, shortness of breath, light-headedness), poor white cell production (infections), and poor platelet production (bruising, prolonged bleeding times).

   Kidney injury is common in multiple myeloma. This can be secondary to hypercalcaemia but also due to deposition of Bence-Jones proteins that are characteristically produced during myeloma and damage the renal tubules.

2. Routine blood tests, checking the full blood count; renal and liver function; and a bone profile should be performed. An erythrocyte sedimentation rate sample should be taken—this is typically elevated in multiple myeloma, as well as other inflammatory conditions. A blood film should be sent to look for features of myelodysplasia.

   Serum and urine protein electrophoresis will confirm the presence of an abnormal paraprotein band (see diagram earlier, which shows serum electrophoresis with the presence of an abnormally raised gamma band). Urine should be sent to look for Bence-Jones proteins (monoclonal globulin protein or immunoglobulin light chains).

   The haematology team will usually perform bone marrow aspiration and trephine sampling. Histological examination of these samples will identify whether abnormal plasma cells are present in the bone marrow to confirm the diagnosis.

3. This patient needs to have his electrolyte imbalances corrected immediately. He will need aggressive fluid rehydration to improve his hypercalcaemia, and if he remains hypercalcaemic after adequate intravenous hydration, then an intravenous bisphosphonate, such as pamidronate, may also be needed to sequester calcium in the bone.

   The patient's blood results show that he has impaired renal function. This may be due to dehydration and hypercalcaemia, but may also be due to renal tubular damage by Bence-Jones protein deposition, as mentioned earlier. Fluid rehydration may help to improve the renal function. Hyperkalaemia can lead to cardiac arrhythmias, and if the potassium level is greater than 6 mmol/L, this should be urgently corrected.

   He will need analgesia for his humeral fracture and a referral to the orthopaedics team.

   Ultimately, a referral to the haematology team will enable a complete investigation and long-term management of this gentleman's multiple myeloma.

   A bone scan is sometimes carried out to identify areas of bone abnormalities, and in this case, there is an abnormal area of myeloma deposition, as indicated by the dark lesion, where the humeral fracture was sustained, as well as in the left radius, left and right tibias, and occiput. Myelomatous deposits show up better on x-rays, and a skeletal survey is usually carried out, where radiographs of the skull, spine, humeri, ribs, pelvis, and femurs are performed.

🔑 KEY POINTS

1. Hypercalcaemia can present with non-specific symptoms such as fatigue, constipation, and joint aches.
2. Fluid rehydration is the key to improving hypercalcaemia in the presence of malignancy. If fluids are not reducing the calcium levels, bisphosphonates, such as pamidronate, can be used.

History

A 68-year-old man has been an inpatient on the stroke unit for several weeks and recently commenced a course of intravenous antibiotics to treat a presumed aspiration pneumonia. He has completed three courses of antibiotics to treat lower respiratory tract infections during his inpatient stay. He has clinically improved, and the consolidation on his chest x-rays is resolving. Prior to discharge, the patient is noted to be febrile and is complaining of new abdominal discomfort. The nurse caring for the patient reports that he has opened his bowels eight times today, passing large volumes of greenish, liquid stool each time.

Examination

The patient looks pale and appears to be in discomfort. His heart sounds are normal, and his chest is clear. The patient's abdomen is distended, generally tender throughout, and the bowel sounds were hyperactive (Figure 7.1).

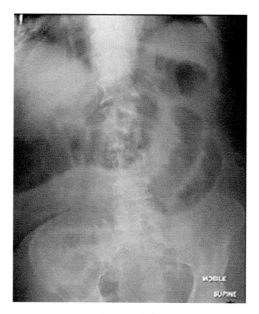

Figure 7.1

Observations: T 38.8°C, HR 108, BP 96/50 mmHg, RR 24, SpO$_2$ 96% on room air

> **? QUESTIONS**
>
> 1. Why may the patient have developed diarrhoea?
> 2. What does the abdominal film show?
> 3. What is the next step in management?

DOI: 10.1201/9781003241171-7

25

ANSWERS

1. The patient has developed profuse diarrhoea following on from a lower respiratory infection that is being treated with multiple antibiotics. The diarrhoea could be related to intolerance of antibiotics or a simple gastrointestinal infection, but in this case, the symptoms and signs seem more concerning. The patient has signs of sepsis (fever, tachycardia, hypotension) and is passing large volumes of liquid stool. In such a case it is important to consider pseudomembranous colitis.

   Clostridium difficile are anaerobic bacteria that can reside in the gut normally, but can also be ingested in institutions such as hospitals and residential homes. When the gut has a normal variety of intestinal flora present, *C. difficile* rarely cause problems. This patient has had multiple courses of antibiotics recently, which will deplete the normal spectrum of bacteria living in the gut. The *C. difficile* bacteria are more likely to survive antibiotic therapy and multiply, over-running the gut. These bacteria release toxins that cause the patient to develop abdominal pain, bloating, and diarrhoea. This leads to symptoms of pseudomembranous colitis. Although any antibiotic can increase the risk of developing a *C. difficile* infection, some are more likely to do so— these include penicillins, fluoroquinolones, and clindamycin.

2. The abdominal film shows prominent, dilated loops of large bowel with evidence of mucosal oedema seen as thickened haustral folds. An x-ray with such an appearance suggests that the patient may have developed toxic megacolon.

3. This patient shows signs of septic shock. Early treatment with intravenous fluid rehydration is necessary. If the patient is not haemodynamically stable, senior help should be sought immediately to consider whether the patient's care needs to be escalated to a critical care unit.

   The microbiology department should be notified of the suspected diagnosis, and stool samples must be sent to look for *C. difficile* toxin. If the patient is well, fluid rehydration may suffice. Sometimes, oral antibiotics targeted at the *C. difficile* bacteria may be needed. Antibiotics that are typically used to treat this infection include metronidazole, vancomycin, and fidaxomicin. Antibiotics to treat pseudomembranous colitis should only be given following microbiologist advice.

   If toxic megacolon (see abdominal x-ray) is suspected, the patient may be at risk of visceral perforation. A nasogastric tube should be sited to allow gastrointestinal decompression, the patient should be made 'nil by mouth', and the surgical team on call will need to review the case.

   Drugs such as loperamide, which slow faecal transit, should be avoided, as these are thought to prolong exposure to the *C. difficile* toxin and worsen the prognosis. Infective spores are present in stool, so effective hand-washing and barrier nursing are necessary to prevent spread of *C. difficile* bacteria among staff and patients. Probiotic drinks taken concurrently with antibiotics may reduce the risk of acquiring *C. difficile* infection, but there is currently no strong evidence to support this.

🔑 KEY POINTS

1. Antibiotics deplete the natural gut flora and place patients at risk of superadded infections by bacteria such as *C. difficile*. You should suspect pseudomembranous colitis in patients who have used antibiotics and present with profuse diarrhoea and other abdominal symptoms.
2. *C. difficile* is highly infective, and proper hand hygiene and barrier nursing should be maintained at all times to prevent further spread of the infection.

CASE 8: WORSENING DELIRIUM

History

An 89-year-old woman has been admitted to hospital with new-onset confusion. The patient's daughter noticed that she had become increasingly forgetful over the past week and now was no longer orientated to time or place. Her past medical history is significant for hypertension, for which she takes 2.5 mg bendroflumethiazide once daily. She is normally independent of activities.

🔎 INVESTIGATIONS

- Her electrolytes and renal function results are shown here. Her urine dip is unremarkable, and her inflammatory markers are not elevated.

	Result	Normal Range
Sodium	114	135–145 mmol/L
Potassium	3.8	3.5–4.5 mmol/L
Urea	6.8	4.0–7.0 mmol/L
Creatinine	98	70–110 mmol/L

Case Progression

The patient is given 4 L of 0.9% saline over the next 24 hours. The following morning, she appears more confused and is now drowsy and dysarthric. When a neurological examination is performed, the patient has reduced power throughout all muscle groups, and there is increased tone and brisk reflexes in the lower limbs. Her blood tests show that her sodium level is now 138 mmol/L.

❓ QUESTIONS

1. What is the probable cause of the lady's initial confusion?
2. Why has the patient deteriorated?

DOI: 10.1201/9781003241171-8

ANSWERS

1. The patient was hyponatraemic at presentation. A sodium level of less than 120 mmol/L indicates severe hyponatraemia. Hyponatraemia is a common electrolyte abnormality and occurs more frequently in elderly patients. Symptoms of hyponatraemia tend to be fairly non-specific and can include nausea, vomiting, and confusion. Serum sodium levels and osmolality are usually tightly controlled by homeostatic mechanisms. As hyponatraemia progresses, patients can develop marked neurological symptoms, such as muscle cramps and seizures, as sodium leaves the bloodstream and the change in osmotic pressures leads to the development of cerebral oedema.

   This patient takes a thiazide diuretic, which acts on the distal convoluted tubule, inhibiting the sodium-chloride symporter so that sodium reabsorption is reduced. This is a common cause of sodium loss in patients. Other drugs that can promote hyponatraemia include loop diuretics, angiotensin-converting enzyme (ACE) inhibitors, selective serotonin reuptake inhibitors, and proton pump inhibitors.

   Patients with any form of fluid overload, such as congestive cardiac failure or nephritic syndrome can develop a hypervolaemic hyponatraemia.

   Hypovolaemic hyponatraemia can occur when patients are losing fluid through vomiting and diarrhoea, not drinking sufficient volumes of water, or becoming volume deplete, for example, due to use of diuretics. Hypovolaemia stimulates antidiuretic hormone (ADH) release and subsequent water retention, which leads to a dilutional hyponatraemia.

   The syndrome of inappropriate ADH release (SIADH) occurs when there is excessive release of ADH, causing water retention and, as stated earlier, a dilutional hyponatraemia. This can be due to damage to the posterior pituitary gland, infections such as meningitis or brain abscesses, and small cell lung cancers that secrete ectopic hormones.

   Determining the patient's fluid status and the underlying cause of the patient's hyponatraemia will help guide management in terms of managing her sodium levels. Measuring urinary sodium levels will inform you as to whether there are abnormalities in tubular reabsorptive function. Paired urine and serum osmolalities will assist you in determining the concentrating ability of the kidneys.

2. The likely diagnosis is that she has developed central pontine myelinolysis. This is a condition that occurs when serum sodium concentrations are rapidly altered, as the osmolar pressures shift, destroying the sensitive myelin sheath around the neurons. Demyelination can lead to severe neurological damage, and the sudden alteration in osmolar pressures can cause cerebral haemorrhage. When treating chronic-onset (>48 hours) hyponatraemia and hypernatraemia, you should aim to correct sodium levels by no more than 8 mmol/L per day. If more rapid correction is needed, this should be done in a closely monitored environment, such as a critical care unit.

🔑 KEY POINTS

1. Hyponatraemia is a common electrolyte abnormality that can cause symptoms of confusion and non-specific malaise. Patients using diuretics should be monitored for hyponatraemia.
2. Rapid correction of hyponatraemia can lead to central pontine myelinolysis—a life-threatening neurological condition.

CASE 9: SWOLLEN GLANDS AND HEARING IMPAIRMENT

History

A 19-year-old medical student has been brought to the emergency department by his flatmates who are concerned that he has become progressively unwell over a period of 5 days. He initially had symptoms of a mild coryzal illness, with a sore throat, headache, and cough. For the past 72 hours he has been intermittently febrile, complaining of right-sided earache and deafness, and nausea. His sore throat is worsening, and he feels as though his "glands are up". He describes struggling to swallow food and fluids due to discomfort around his throat. He has no significant past medical history and did not experience any significant childhood illnesses, although he did not receive all of his childhood vaccinations due to parental concerns regarding immunisation.

Examination

This young man is febrile (T 38.7°C) and tachycardic with a heart rate of 112 beats per minute. His heart sounds are normal, and his chest is clear. His abdomen is soft and non-tender. There is marked bilateral cervical lymphadenopathy, and his right ear is erythematous and swollen. He has painful bilateral testicular swelling.

 INVESTIGATIONS

- Routine blood tests show elevated inflammatory markers, normal renal function, and normal liver function. An HIV test was negative.
- An audiogram shows significant hearing loss in the left ear (Figure 9.1): the straight line represents normal hearing at particular frequencies, and anything below this would be classed as abnormal.

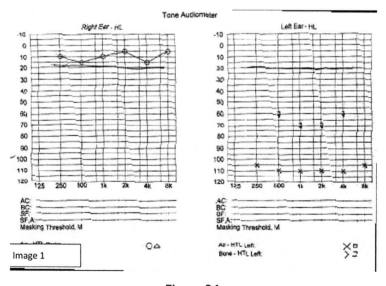

Figure 9.1

DOI: 10.1201/9781003241171-9

1. What condition does this young man have?
2. How would you treat the patient?

ANSWERS

1. The patient has mumps, which is a viral illness. Patients typically develop painful swelling of the parotid glands, which initially starts as a sore throat and can progress to odynophagia (pain on swallowing). The illness is often mild and self-limiting in younger children but tends to be more severe in teenagers and adults. As well as parotitis, patients may complain of headache, fevers, and orchitis. Around 30% of males will develop orchitis, and half of these will be left with minor testicular atrophy. Rarely, post-pubescent males can be left infertile as a result of prolonged orchitis.

   Although occurring less frequently than other symptoms, hearing loss can be one of the more serious consequences of mumps infection. Mumps is the most common cause of unilateral acquired sensorineural hearing loss in children and young adults worldwide, so physicians should advise patients with a suspected mumps infection to report any changes in their hearing. Occasionally, the disease can progress to encephalitis, but this is very uncommon.

   The incubation period for mumps is usually 14–18 days from exposure to onset of symptoms. The infectious period is from 3 days before until approximately 9 days after onset of symptoms. The more serious complications of mumps, such as meningitis, encephalitis, and orchitis, may occur in the absence of parotitis, which can delay accurate diagnosis of the clinical syndrome.

   Outbreaks remain frequent, particularly among students. As uptake in the measles, mumps, rubella (MMR) vaccination programme has fallen in many areas over recent years, diseases like measles and mumps are becoming increasingly common.

2. Treatment is primarily supportive, so symptoms of pain are controlled with analgesia, and fevers are treated with paracetamol. If there is evidence of hearing impairment, oral steroids should be started urgently. This patient complained of hearing loss, and an audiogram was performed, which showed that he had left-sided sensorineural deafness as a result of his infection.

1. Mumps infections are becoming increasingly common in many areas, particularly following reduced uptake of the MMR vaccine over the past 15 years.
2. Suspect mumps in a patient who presents with parotitis and fevers.
3. Patients should be made aware that hearing loss can occur as a result of mumps infection and to be vigilant for any symptoms. Start steroid therapy if there are any signs or symptoms of sensorineural hearing loss.

CASE 10: NOSE BLEED (EPISTAXIS) FOLLOWING AN OPERATION

History

An 85-year-old woman presents to hospital following a fall down the stairs at home. She has fractured her left neck of the femur and has been admitted to the orthopaedic ward. Her past medical history includes hypertension and chronic renal impairment, with a baseline estimated glomerular filtration rate of 50 mL/min/1.73m^2.

The patient undergoes a successful surgical reduction and internal fixation and initially appears well post-operatively, although she does develop a right-sided lower limb deep vein thrombosis (DVT). The surgical team prescribe a daily therapeutic dose of low-molecular-weight heparin to treat the DVT. Four days later, the patient complains that she has a nosebleed for over 30 minutes.

INVESTIGATIONS

- The patient's full blood count at admission was WCC 9.9, Hb 12.4, Plt 350.
- A repeat full blood count was taken after the nosebleed: WCC 10.6, Hb 10.8, Plt 90.

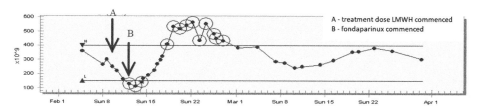

Figure 10.1 Graph to show platelet levels during admission.

QUESTIONS

1. Why might the patient's platelet count be falling?
2. Should you stop the heparin?

DOI: 10.1201/9781003241171-10

ANSWERS

1. This woman needs to be investigated for heparin-induced thrombocytopaenia (HIT). This is a condition that typically develops 4–10 days after commencing treatment with heparin and is more common with unfractionated heparin rather than LMWH. IgG antibodies to heparin develop that activate platelets and cause clot formation. This causes the platelet count to fall and also predisposes patients to thrombosis.

   A HIT screen can be performed, sending blood samples for an enzyme-linked immunosorbent assay (ELISA) test to identify heparin-binding antibodies. Doppler ultrasound scans of the legs tend to be performed routinely in anyone suspected of having HIT, as DVTs are very common in this condition. The graph provided shows the patient's platelet count during her hospital stay.

2. Patients with HIT have a low circulating platelet count, which can predispose them to bleeding, but they paradoxically have an increased risk of thrombosis due to platelet activation. The heparin should be ceased, but ongoing anticoagulation is required to prevent clot formation. Warfarin is contraindicated, as patients with HIT are predisposed to warfarin-related necrosis. The haematology team should be contacted to provide advice regarding ongoing anticoagulation. There are numerous options available, including danaparoid, which is a low-molecular-weight heparinoid devoid of heparin, and fondaparinux, which is a synthetic anticoagulant that inhibits factor Xa but does not inhibit thrombin.

 KEY POINTS

1. HIT is the development of thrombocytopaenia following treatment with heparin and typically presents 4–10 days after the first dose.
2. HIT predisposes to thrombosis, and treatment requires anticoagulation with an agent that will not further reduce the platelet count.

CASE 11: DELIBERATE SELF-HARM WITH ANTIFREEZE

History

A 32-year-old man is brought to hospital by ambulance having been found collapsed in bed at home. The paramedics report that they found an opened bottle of antifreeze in his bedroom; the label specified that the product contained greater than 50% ethylene glycol. There were no empty tablet packets or signs of alcohol consumption in the room. The patient has a past medical history of depression and emotionally unstable personality disorder, with several previous admissions to hospital with deliberate self-harm. He has been prescribed sertraline 100 mg OD but has not collected his prescription for several months. He lives with two flatmates and works as a waiter in a restaurant. He does not smoke, and his flatmates report that he does not drink alcohol regularly.

Examination

The patient is drowsy but responsive to pain. He is afebrile. Cardiovascular, respiratory, and abdominal examinations are unremarkable. Neurological examination is challenging due to the patient's reduced level of consciousness; however, there are no obvious cranial nerve deficits, and the limbs have normal tone and reflexes throughout.

🔍 INVESTIGATIONS

An ABG taken on room air showed:

- pH: 7.06
- pO_2: 12.0 kPa
- pCO_2: 2.7 kPa
- Sodium: 140 mmols
- Potassium: 4.0 mmols
- Chloride: 103 mmol/L
- Bicarbonate (standard): 8 mmol/L
- Base excess: −26
- Lactate: 4.4 mmol/L
- Blood glucose level: 4.5 mmol/L
- Blood ketone level: 1.9 mmol/L
- Paracetamol level: undetectable
- Salicylate level: undetectable

❓ QUESTIONS

1. Interpret the blood gas.
2. How should this patient be managed acutely?

DOI: 10.1201/9781003241171-11

ANSWERS

1. This patient has an acidosis, as evidenced by the low pH. The bicarbonate level and base excess are reduced, indicating that this is a metabolic acidosis. The low carbon dioxide level indicates that partial respiratory compensation has occurred.

   The anion gap can be calculated by subtracting the primary measured anions (bicarbonate and chloride) from the primary measured cation (sodium). In this case, the result is 29 mmol/L (reference range 3–11 mmol/L).

   The causes of an elevated anion gap metabolic acidosis include ketoacidosis (this patient has a mildly raised ketone level), salicylate and paracetamol toxicity, uraemia, lactic acidosis, and alcohol/toxic alcohol poisoning.

2. In this case, it is likely that the patient has ingested ethylene glycol, and blood samples should be taken at presentation to measure serum ethylene glycol levels. In cases of self-poisoning, paracetamol and salicylate levels should also be sent if the patient could have had access to these. If paracetamol overdose is suspected, treatment with N-acetylcysteine may be indicated.

   The patient should be treated with fomepizole, a competitive inhibitor of the alcohol dehydrogenase enzyme, to slow the production of toxic ethylene glycol metabolites (glycolate and oxalate). Alternatively, ethanol can be used to inhibit alcohol dehydrogenase if fomepizole is not available. The patient should also receive intravenous sodium bicarbonate to treat the metabolic acidosis as well as general supportive care. Haemodialysis may be required in patients with a persistent metabolic acidosis, deranged electrolytes, or haemodynamic instability. The emergency department team should access local or national expert toxicology advice where available.

🔑 KEY POINTS

1. Ethylene glycol toxicity is one of the causes of a raised anion gap metabolic acidosis. Other causes include ketoacidosis, salicylate and paracetamol toxicity, and a lactic acidosis.
2. Toxic alcohol ingestion may be managed with fomepizole, a competitive inhibitor of the alcohol dehydrogenase enzyme. Always seek expert toxicology advice (where available) when managing patients with toxic alcohol poisoning.

CASE 12: RIGHT-SIDED CHEST PAIN

History

A 38-year-old woman presents to the emergency department complaining of chest pain and shortness of breath. The pain is sharp in nature, is located around the right side of her chest, and becomes worse on deep inspiration. Both the chest pain and the shortness of breath developed over the course of 1–2 hours. The patient denies any symptoms of cough or fever. Her past medical history is significant for two miscarriages and a previous deep vein thrombosis (DVT) in her left calf. Aside from the combined oral contraceptive pill, she does not take any regular medications. The patient's mother and sister have also both experienced DVTs. She works as a shop assistant, has never smoked, and drinks approximately 10 units of alcohol per week.

Examination

The patient appears comfortable at rest. There is good air entry throughout the lung fields, and the chest is clear to auscultation. The heart sounds are normal. Her abdomen is soft and non-tender. Her calves are soft and non-tender, and there is no peripheral oedema.

Observations

Heart rate: 94 beats per minute, blood pressure: 126/82 mmHg, respiratory rate: 20 breaths per minute, SpO$_2$: 93% on room air.

🔍 INVESTIGATIONS

- WCC 5.6
- Hb 128
- Plt 163
- Na 140
- K 4.5
- Creat 68
- CRP 5
- D-dimer 2.17
- Chest x-ray—clear lung fields, no focal consolidation

? QUESTIONS

1. What is the differential diagnosis?
2. How would you further investigate and manage the patient?

DOI: 10.1201/9781003241171-12

ANSWERS

1. The patient has pleuritic chest pain with shortness of breath.

   This could be a pneumonia, although you would typically expect symptoms of a cough or fever plus abnormal findings such as coarse crackles on auscultation of the chest. Additionally, the patient does not have raised inflammatory markers, and her chest x-ray is unremarkable.

   A pneumothorax can cause pleuritic chest pain and shortness of breath, but you would expect to hear reduced or absent breath sounds at the site of the pneumothorax, and the chest x-ray would also show this.

   Musculoskeletal injuries can cause chest pain that is worsened by deep inspiration or moving in general. In this case, the patient gives no history of any exercise or trauma preceding the pain, and her oxygen saturations are reduced, which would not be expected with musculoskeletal chest pain.

   Based on the patient's symptoms of shortness of breath and pleuritic chest pain, plus the low oxygen saturations, a pulmonary embolus (PE) is the most likely diagnosis. Risk factors for PEs include:

   - Prolonged immobility, such as after surgery or a long-haul flight
   - Pregnancy
   - Use of oestrogen-containing medication, such as the oral contraceptive pill
   - Malignancy
   - Thrombophilias, such as factor V Leiden and antiphospholipid syndrome

   PEs are usually preceded by a DVT. This patient has previously had a DVT, as have her mother and sister, suggesting a genetic cause for her clot. The patient has also had multiple miscarriages. She may have antiphospholipid syndrome, a prothrombotic condition that predisposes patients to arterial and venous blood clots, that classically presents with a combination of DVTs, PEs, and miscarriages. The patient also takes the combined oral contraceptive pill, which further increases her risk of developing clots.

2. If you suspect that the patient has a PE, you can calculate her Wells score to guide your decision to further investigate this. The Wells score is a clinical prediction rule that enables the user to calculate the likelihood of their patient having a PE based on certain clinical criteria. A score of 0–1 equates to a low probability for a PE, while a score of 2–6 equates to an intermediate probability for a PE. A score of 7 or more indicates that the patient has a high risk for a PE.

   A D-dimer blood test can also be performed to help guide the diagnosis when there is a low probability for a PE. D-dimer is a fibrin degradation product that can form in the presence of a large blood clot, but can also form with most causes of inflammation, such as an injury, an infection, or malignancy. An elevated serum D-dimer level does not confirm that the patient has a PE, but a normal D-dimer level will exclude a PE in the vast majority of cases. In this case, the patient has a markedly elevated D-dimer level with no corresponding rise in inflammatory markers and no other obvious reason for it to be high aside from a PE.

   As this patient has low oxygen saturations, an arterial blood gas should be performed to assess for hypoxia, and oxygen therapy should be given if necessary. Provided that there are no contraindications to anticoagulation, either a direct oral anticoagulant, such as rivaroxaban, or a low-molecular-weight heparin (LMWH), such as dalteparin, should be commenced whilst the patient awaits further imaging.

Either a ventilation-perfusion (VQ) scan or a CT scan of the pulmonary arteries (CTPA) should be performed to assess for the presence of a PE.

If the patient does indeed have a PE, long-term anticoagulation should be given for at least 3 months, and they should be followed up in an anticoagulation clinic where further investigations can be considered. This patient has several features of antiphospholipid syndrome and should therefore be investigated further for this condition with blood tests for anticardiolipin IgG and lupus anticoagulant at a later date. Any of the previous risk factors for PE should be minimised.

KEY POINTS

1. Consider a PE in a patient with pleuritic chest pain, shortness of breath, or haemoptysis, particularly if they have any of the risk factors noted earlier.
2. A Wells score can help in deciding whether the patient is at low, moderate, or high risk for developing a PE.
3. A D-dimer test can be performed and is useful in excluding a PE if the levels are normal. A high D-dimer does not mean that the patient has a PE, but rather that there is some active inflammation.

CASE 13: A CASE OF DELIBERATE SELF-HARM

History

A 19-year-old student is admitted to hospital after being found unconscious in her room in the university halls of residence. Her roommate told the paramedics that the patient had recently failed her end-of-year exams. She is not known to have any previous medical history and only takes occasional painkillers for a knee injury. The patient was reportedly found with several packets of paracetamol and codeine phosphate nearby and an empty bottle of wine on her bedside table. The patient is now awake and conscious and admits to taking an unspecified number of tablets approximately 4 hours earlier. She complains of nausea and has vomited several times.

Examination

The patient's observations were T 36.4 °C, HR 80 bpm, BP 110/70 mmHg, RR 12, SaO_2 96% on room air. On examination, she was drowsy but responsive to voice. Her heart sounds are normal, and her chest is clear. There is some mild epigastric tenderness present. A full neurological examination is unremarkable.

Results

Blood tests:

WCC 7.0, Hb 12.6, Plt 290, Na 139, K 4.9, creat 75, CRP <5, bili 20, ALT 35, ALP 43, alb 45, INR 1.1

? QUESTIONS

1. The patient has taken a paracetamol overdose—what consequences can this have?
2. How would you manage this patient's care?

DOI: 10.1201/9781003241171-13

ANSWERS

1. Paracetamol overdose is the leading cause of acute liver failure in the United Kingdom. Paracetamol overdose can lead to the accumulation of N-acetyl-p- benzoquinoneimine (NAPQI), a toxic intermediate metabolite that causes cytotoxic effects. Glutathione is an antioxidant that conjugates with NAPQI to produce non-toxic metabolites. In the case of paracetamol overdose, the glutathione stores can become depleted, leading to accumulation of NAPQI and subsequent hepatocellular damage.

   Liver failure can develop over hours, or even days. In this case, the patient has also taken opioid medication (codeine phosphate) alongside alcohol, both of which may further impair hepatic function.

2. In most centres, activated charcoal will be given if the patient presents within an hour of taking the overdose. This is a highly porous substance and can adsorb substances such as paracetamol, thus preventing further metabolism of these toxins.

   A 4-hour serum paracetamol level should be taken, and the results of this test should be plotted on a paracetamol toxicity nomogram (Figure 13.1) to guide further treatment. If the patient's paracetamol level is above or within 10% of the treatment line, a course of N-acetylcysteine therapy should be commenced.

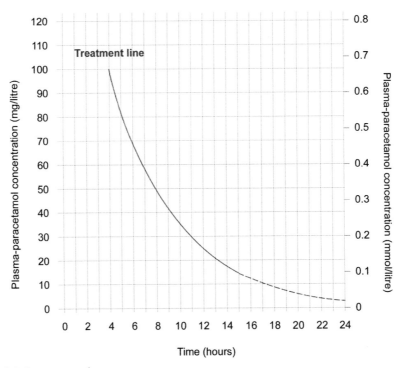

Figure 13.1 Paracetamol treatment normogram.

(*Source:* Image from Royal College of Emergency Medicine Guidance, www.rcem.ac.uk/RCEM/Quality-Policy/Clinical_Standards_Guidance/RCEM_Guidance.aspx?WebsiteKey=b3d6bb2a-abba-44ed-b758-467776a958cd&hkey=862bd964-0363-4f7f-bdab-89e4a68c9de4&RCEM_Guidance=6)

Blood tests should be sent to monitor the liver function, and early results may show a hepatitic picture with raised transaminases. Liver synthetic function should be monitored closely. The liver produces coagulation factors, and measuring the international normalised ratio (INR) will indicate how effective the liver is at synthesising these products. Renal function should also be closely monitored, as an acute kidney injury can also occur.

After 3–5 days, patients are at risk of hepatic necrosis. Patients can present with sepsis, impaired clotting function, and multi-organ failure.

Patients should have regular observations, and blood tests (liver function, renal function, and coagulation screen) should be monitored. In addition to the aforementioned blood tests, blood glucose checks may need to be performed, as patients can become hypoglycaemic in liver failure.

The mainstay of treatment is N-acetylcysteine, which replenishes the stores of glutathione and prevents further liver damage. This treatment is very effective at preventing hepatocellular damage, particularly if given within 8 hours of the overdose. For patients who develop fulminant hepatic failure, a liver transplant may be necessary.

In the longer term, the patient should have a psychiatric review to assess her risk of ongoing self-harm and to consider implementing further support in the community.

🔑 KEY POINTS

1. Paracetamol overdose is the leading cause of liver failure in the United Kingdom.
2. Patients should be treated with fluids and may require N-acetylcysteine therapy depending on their serum paracetamol concentrations and the timing of the overdose.
3. In severe toxicity, hepatic failure may develop, particularly if the patient presents to hospital more than 8 hours after the overdose occurred. A liver transplant may be considered in severe cases.

CASE 14: LYMPHADENOPATHY AND MALAISE

History

A 19-year-old woman has presented to the emergency department complaining of fevers and general malaise. Over the preceding 3–4 days, she noticed a rash develop over her trunk and limbs. She also complains of a sore throat and feels very fatigued. She has no significant past history and does not take any regular medications or recreational drugs. She does not smoke, nor drink alcohol. She states that she has had several episodes of unprotected sexual intercourse with a male partner that she recently met. There is no recent travel history.

Examination

The patient is febrile (38.0°C) and tachycardic with a heart rate of 106 beats per minute. Her heart sounds are normal, her chest is clear, and her abdomen is soft and non-tender. She has palpable cervical and axillary lymphadenopathy: the lymph nodes are 15–20 mm and soft and tender on palpation. There is an erythematous, maculopapular rash covering her trunk, upper arms, and thighs.

INVESTIGATIONS

Blood test	Results
White cells	14.0
Haemoglobin	15.0
Platelets	100
Sodium	133
Potassium	3.7
Urea	4.5
Creatinine	77
CRP	78

QUESTIONS

1. What are the possible diagnoses that you should consider?
2. If the HIV test is positive, how will you proceed?

DOI: 10.1201/9781003241171-14

ANSWERS

1. This woman is likely to have a viral illness, considering her history of fevers, rash, and sore throat.

   Infectious mononucleosis (glandular fever) secondary to Epstein-Barr virus is a common illness in young adults, presenting with fever, rash, and lymphadenopathy following on from a sore throat. A Monospot antibody test can rapidly identify patients with current Epstein-Barr infections. Blood tests typically show a lymphocytosis and possibly an acute hepatitis, from which patients will gradually recover over the following weeks.

   In the winter months, influenza is a common viral infection that affects people of all ages.

   HIV is another infection that must be considered, particularly if the patient reports risk factors, such as intravenous drug use or unprotected sexual intercourse. The patient should be advised to undergo an HIV test, and the health care professional that counsels her for this should also explain that it can take up to 6 weeks postexposure for the HIV test to become positive (seroconversion). HIV seroconversion typically presents as a short-lived illness with headache, fever, sore throat, and rash that occurs within 6 weeks of the exposure event.

   If the HIV test is currently negative, then the patient should have a repeat test 6 weeks later—this can be arranged at a local sexual health clinic.

   In areas with a high HIV prevalence, HIV screening is often carried out routinely when a patient presents to a hospital or other health care facility, regardless of their reason for attending. HIV screening successfully identifies patients with HIV who may not have otherwise been diagnosed until many months or years later.

2. If the patient has a positive HIV test, in addition to the full blood count, blood samples should be sent to measure the CD4 and CD8 counts and the HIV viral load, as well as the renal and hepatic function.

   T lymphocytes express either CD4 molecules, which initiate an immune response to bacteria, viruses, and fungi, or CD8 molecules. The HIV virus binds to CD4 molecules and rapidly reproduces. As patients seroconvert in the weeks following infection, they develop symptoms consistent with a viral illness, such as fevers and lymphadenopathy.

   The CD4 cells are gradually destroyed by the virus, and after several years, patients begin to develop opportunistic infections.

   The patient should be referred to the local HIV team who can take a focused history and identify any specific treatment that she will need, such as antiretroviral medication to treat the HIV infection. She should undergo testing for other sexually transmitted infections, such as syphilis, gonorrhoea, and chlamydia. Contact tracing should also be encouraged, so that anyone else at risk of contracting HIV from the patient, or the person who passed the infection to the patient, can be identified.

🔑 KEY POINTS

1. Consider HIV infection in patients presenting with symptoms such as fever, rash, lymphadenopathy, or arthropathy.
2. Patients with a positive HIV test should be referred to an HIV team who can monitor CD4 counts and commence appropriate antiretroviral therapy.

CASE 15: LOSS OF CONSCIOUSNESS IN DIABETES

A 16-year-old girl was found unconscious in her room and has been brought to hospital. She was diagnosed with type 1 diabetes mellitus 3 years earlier and currently uses NovoMix 30 (a biphasic insulin analogue), 12 units twice daily. Her glycated haemoglobin (HbA1c) level was checked last month and was reportedly elevated, indicating poor control of her blood glucose levels over the preceding 3 months. The patient has been suffering from a sore throat and influenza-like symptoms over the past 2–3 days. Her parents report that she had administered lower doses of insulin in the past 48 hours, as her appetite has been poor and she has eaten less food than normal.

Examination

The patient's mucous membranes were dry, and her abdomen was soft but tender throughout. She vomits several times during the examination. She appears short of breath and is gasping.

Her capillary blood glucose level, checked by the paramedics, is 24 mmol/L.

Observations: temperature 36.8 °C, HR 110 bpm, BP 90/50 mmHg, RR 32, SaO$_2$ 99% on room air.

INVESTIGATIONS

- Urine dip: 4+ glucose, 3+ ketones.
- Arterial blood gas sample taken on room air: pH 7.12, pO$_2$ 12.8, pCO$_2$ 2.8, lactate 4.0, HCO$_3$ 18, base excess −6

QUESTIONS

1. What is the underlying diagnosis?
2. How would you manage this patient acutely?

DOI: 10.1201/9781003241171-15

ANSWERS

1. The patient has diabetic ketoacidosis (DKA). She has not been adhering to her usual insulin regimen and is now hyperglycaemic. She has ketones in her urine, and the blood gas sample shows a metabolic acidosis (low pH with low HCO3; the pCO_2 is also low, ruling out any respiratory component to the acidosis).

   The criteria for DKA include:

   a. Hyperglycaemia (blood glucose >11 mmol/L)

   b. Ketosis: plasma ketones >3 mmol/L and/or urinary ketones ≥2+

   c. Acidosis: pH <7.35

   When people become dehydrated, the body produces stress hormones that increase glucose availability to allow for increased metabolic requirements. When there is a lack of insulin in the body, such as in this case, high levels of glucose are released by the liver from glycogen stores and gluconeogenesis. The kidneys begin to excrete glucose in the urine and an osmotic diuresis occurs; this leads to water and electrolytes leaving the body in the urine. The patient experiences polyuria and becomes increasingly dehydrated. Fatty acids are broken down, producing ketones.

2. The patient is likely to be severely dehydrated. The priority should be to correct her fluid status, as this is more dangerous than the hyperglycaemia. Patients typically have a fluid deficit of 100 mL/kg or more. Most hospitals will have a local protocol to guide management of DKA. Fluid balance should be carefully monitored with a fluid input/output chart updated hourly. A urinary catheter may need to be inserted to monitor urine output.

   Patients who have signs of sepsis (fever, SBP <100 mmHg, HR >100), are drowsy or confused, or who have a severe acidosis (pH <7.10) may need to be managed on a critical care unit. All children and most young adults (20 years of age or younger) should also be managed on a critical care unit, as they are at greater risk of developing cerebral oedema in response to shifts in osmolarity.

   A typical treatment regimen involves administering 500 mL 0.9% sodium chloride over 15 minutes, followed by 1000 mL 0.9% saline over 2 hours. This second bag of fluid should contain 20 mmol potassium chloride unless the patient has a serum potassium level of >5 mmol/L (reference range 3.5–5.0 mmol/L). This is because patients with DKA often have a significant intracellular potassium deficit, and the potassium levels will fall further once intravenous fluids and insulin are commenced.

   An intravenous fixed-rate insulin infusion that is adjusted based on results of hourly capillary blood glucose levels should be commenced at this point. This uses a fast-acting insulin, such as Actrapid, with the aim of reducing the blood glucose by 3–5 mmol/L/hour until the target glucose level of 12–18 mmol/L has been reached. Intravenous fluids (0.9% sodium chloride +/– potassium chloride) should continue. The acidosis will usually resolve with fluid rehydration and correction of hyperglycaemia. As the insulin levels increase, fatty acid breakdown will cease and ketones will no longer be produced. Usually, once glucose levels fall to 18 mmol/L, an intravenous glucose infusion is prescribed (e.g. 10% 500 mL over 8 hours).

   After 24 hours of treatment, if patients have urinary ketones of 0 to +1 or plasma ketone levels of <0.3 mmol/L and are tolerating food and oral fluids, then they can revert back to their usual subcutaneous insulin regimen.

Following resolution of DKA, the patient should be educated, ideally by a diabetes nurse specialist, about the importance of maintaining adequate hydration and regular blood glucose monitoring at home to allow insulin to be titrated accordingly.

🔑 KEY POINTS

1. DKA is a life-threatening condition and should be treated urgently. The priority is to rehydrate the patient, then correct the high glucose levels. You may also need to replace potassium deficits. Patients will need close monitoring of their blood glucose and acid-base status in addition to their hydration status.
2. There should be a low threshold for referring children, young adults, and patients with signs of sepsis or severe acidosis for admission to a critical care unit.

CASE 16: FEVERS, WEIGHT LOSS, AND NIGHT SWEATS

History

A 54-year-old woman presents to the emergency department with a 2-week history of fevers and night sweats. She denies experiencing shortness of breath, cough, or haemoptysis but she had been feeling very fatigued and had a poor appetite. Although she has not weighed herself recently, her clothes feel loose, and she suspects that she has unintentionally lost 4–5 kg in weight over this time. There is no significant past medical history, drug history, or family history. The patient has not travelled abroad in the last 5 years and has no known tuberculosis contacts. She has never smoked and does not drink alcohol. She works in an administrative job.

Examination

The patient appears comfortable at rest. She is afebrile. Her heart sounds are normal, her chest is clear, and her abdomen is soft and non-tender. Of note, there is palpable cervical, axillary, and inguinal lymphadenopathy. The lymph nodes are 2–3 cm in diameter and feel rubbery.

Results

A chest x-ray was performed (see Figure 16.1).

A lymph node biopsy confirms that the patient has a non-Hodgkin's lymphoma.

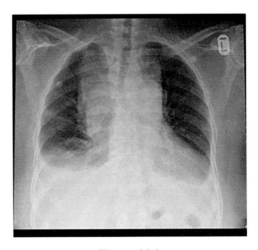

Figure 16.1

Case Progression

The patient commences her first course of chemotherapy and tolerates this well. Five days after completing the first course, however, she presents to the emergency department complaining of fevers and a cough productive of yellow sputum. She is found to have a fever of 40.2°C. Her full blood count is as follows:

Blood Test	Result	Reference Range
White cells	2.9	$4–11 \times 10^9$/L
Neutrophils	0.5	$2–7 \times 10^9$/L
Haemoglobin	110	120–160 g/L
Platelets	154	$150–400 \times 10^9$/L

DOI: 10.1201/9781003241171-16

? QUESTIONS

1. What does the chest x-ray show, and what is the differential diagnosis for such an appearance?
2. What condition has she developed as a result of her chemotherapy?

ANSWERS

1. The chest x-ray shows a widened mediastinum, as well as bilateral pleural effusions and some middle lobe shadowing. The hila are bulky bilaterally due to lymphadenopathy. Several disease processes can cause this appearance, including:

   - Primary lung malignancy
   - Malignancy with lung metastases
   - Lymphoma
   - Tuberculosis
   - Sarcoidosis

2. The patient has presented with a febrile neutropenia (also known as neutropenic sepsis). The chemotherapy has suppressed her bone marrow function, and she now has a very low neutrophil count, which puts her at high risk of bacterial infections.

   She will need to commence antibiotics for neutropenic sepsis as per the antibiotic protocol of the individual hospital. She should ideally receive the antibiotics within an hour, as per the Surviving Sepsis Campaign guidelines (www.survivingsepsis.org). Samples of blood, urine, sputum, and stool should be sent for microscopy, culture, and sensitivity to attempt to isolate a specific bacterium causing the infection.

   The patient's blood count will need to be monitored at least once per day. Bone marrow suppression can also lead to reduced red cell and platelet counts. The haematology team will need to review the patient and may consider giving granulocyte colony-stimulating factor (gCSF) to improve bone marrow function.

   She should be nursed in a side room, and barrier protection (face masks, gloves, and aprons) should be worn when coming into contact with the patient to prevent introducing further sources of infection.

🔑 KEY POINTS

1. Chemotherapy can suppress the bone marrow, leading to pancytopaenia. A low neutrophil count in patients on chemotherapy is strongly associated with increased risk of developing bacterial infections.
2. Neutropenic sepsis is a medical emergency and requires urgent treatment with antibiotics.

CASE 17: THE ILL RETURNING TRAVELLER

History

A 46-year-old man has presented to the emergency department complaining of fevers, vomiting, and general malaise. He reports having experienced fevers and rigors every 8–12 hours for the past 3 days. He feels weak and tired and has vomited several times. He describes some mild abdominal discomfort but denies diarrhoea or constipation. He is usually fit and well with no past medical history and takes no regular medications. The patient works in an office, smokes five cigarettes daily, and drinks approximately 10 units of alcohol per week. He has recently returned from a holiday in Ghana where he took part in a camping trip.

Examination

The patient appears pale, and his mucous membranes are dry. He is febrile (39.7°C) and tachycardic (100 beats per minute). His abdomen is soft throughout but tender at the left upper quadrant, where splenomegaly of approximately 8 cm is palpable. There is no cervical, axillary, or inguinal lymphadenopathy. The patient has multiple excoriated lesions around his ankles, which he attributes to mosquito bites.

? **QUESTIONS**

1. Considering the possible diagnosis, which investigations should you send?
2. How should this man be treated?

ANSWERS

1. The patient describes swinging pyrexias and has moderate splenomegaly. He has recently returned from Ghana and has visible mosquito bites on his extremities. It is not clear from the history whether or not the patient took antimalarial prophylaxis. The clinical features fit a diagnosis of malaria, and appropriate tests should be sent to look for this.

   A full blood count may show an anaemia (predominantly due to red blood cells being destroyed by malaria parasites) and a thrombocytopaenia. Renal and liver function may also be deranged. A blood film will confirm the presence of malaria parasites in addition to identifying the species of parasite and measuring blood parasite levels.

2. The treatment will depend on which type of malaria the patient has—until this is established, patients should be treated as for falciparum malaria with quinine, atovaquone with proguanil hydrochloride, or artemether with lumefantrine.

   Plasmodium falciparum infection with a high parasite count will need initial treatment with intravenous quinine. An intravenous 5% glucose infusion may also need to be given, as blood glucose levels can fall as a result of numerous processes, including increased glucose requirements due to fever and infection, as well as glucose consumption by the malaria parasites. Other types of malaria, such as *Plasmodium malariae*, *Plasmodium vivax*, and *Plasmodium ovale*, are more benign and can usually be managed with a short course of oral antimalarials.

 KEY POINTS

1. Malaria should be suspected in patients with an appropriate travel history who present with fevers and rigors.
2. In patients with suspected malaria, blood should be sent for blood films, looking for the presence of the parasites.
3. Once a parasite has been identified, treatment advice can be sought from an infectious diseases specialist to guide further management.

CASE 18: AN ATYPICAL SEIZURE

History

A 28-year-old woman has been brought by ambulance to the emergency department after she experienced an episode of collapse followed by violent thrashing movements of her arms and legs whilst she was at work. The patient has had a second episode in hospital, which was witnessed by staff. She was seen to become suddenly unresponsive with jerking of her limbs. She resisted eye opening and was breathing rapidly. There was no tongue biting or urinary incontinence. The patient became fully alert within 30 seconds of the episode and has remained well since. She reports no significant past medical history and takes no regular medications. She describes being well over recent weeks and has no unwell contacts. She does not drink alcohol and has never smoked.

Examination

Systemic examination, including a full neurological assessment was unremarkable.

 INVESTIGATIONS

- An ECG showed normal sinus rhythm with a rate of 70 beats per minute.
- Full blood count, renal profile, and CRP—all within the reference ranges.
- Venous blood gas pH 7.40, sodium 137 mmol/L, potassium 4.0 mmol/L, glucose 4.4 mmol/L, lactate 0.8 mmol/L.
- A CT scan of the brain showed no intracranial pathology.
- An EEG showed normal brain activity.

? QUESTIONS

1. What is the likely diagnosis?
2. How should the condition be managed?

DOI: 10.1201/9781003241171-18

ANSWERS

1. In view of the patient's presentation, it is likely that she is experiencing non-epileptic seizures. The majority of psychogenic seizures are dissociative in nature, meaning that the episode may happen as a subconscious attempt to prevent traumatic thoughts, and the patient is unable to control the episodes.

   Although there are no features that definitively separate epileptic and dissociative seizures, it is worth noting that it is uncommon for epileptic seizures to last for more than 5 minutes, whilst this occurs more frequently with dissociative seizures. Tongue biting, urinary incontinence, significant injuries, and an elevated lactate level are more likely to indicate an epileptic seizure rather than a dissociative one. Side-to-side head movements, thrashing movements, and forced closure of the eyes and mouth can also signify a dissociative seizure.

2. Dissociative seizures are diagnosed once other causes for the episodes, such as epilepsy, cardiogenic or metabolic conditions, and structural brain abnormalities, have been excluded. A typical work-up includes blood tests, an ECG, a brain scan (CT or MRI), and an EEG.

   Patients benefit from a positive diagnosis rather than simply being told that they do not have epilepsy or have 'non-epileptic seizures'. It is also important to emphasise to patients that their condition is genuine and not an imagined or faked problem. Treatments may include cognitive behaviour therapy, counselling, psychotherapy, and input from specialist neurology and neuropsychiatry teams.

 KEY POINTS

1. It can be challenging to differentiate between epileptic and psychogenic seizures, but the presence of certain features, such as side-to-side head movements, thrashing movements, and forced closure of the eyes, are more common in the latter.
2. Patients with dissociative seizures benefit from being given a positive diagnosis, rather than an explanation of the diseases in terms of epilepsy. Support via cognitive behavioural therapy and neuropsychiatry specialist input may be beneficial.

CASE 19: DELIRIUM AND URINARY SYMPTOMS

History

An 88-year-old woman has been admitted to hospital after her daughter visited and found her to be confused. For the past 3 days, the patient had complained of feeling tired and had become increasingly disorientated. She is normally relatively fit and well. On direct questioning, the patient describes symptoms of urinary frequency and dysuria. Her past medical history includes osteoarthritis, and she takes paracetamol for this as needed. She lives alone and is independent with all activities of daily living. She smokes four cigarettes daily and drinks 15 units of alcohol per week.

Examination

The patient is febrile (T 39.4°C) and tachycardic (108 beats per minute). She is a slim lady, weighing approximately 55 kg. Her heart sounds are normal, and her chest is clear. Her abdomen is soft with mild suprapubic tenderness. The neurological examination is unremarkable. Her abbreviated mental test score is 6/10.

🔍 INVESTIGATIONS

- Urine dip: 3+ leucocytes, nitrites positive
- Blood tests: WCC 18.0, neutrophils 16.0, Hb 130, Plt 305, Na 138, K 3.9, urea 12.0, creat 140, CRP 94

? QUESTIONS

1. What is the likely underlying cause of this patient's confusion?
2. Over the first few hours the patient remains tachycardic (heart rate 100 bpm) and her blood pressure falls to 100/70 mmHg. What should be done?
3. Her heart rate remains high despite initial treatment, and her blood pressure continues to fall (70/30 mmHg). Her urine output is initially good (60 mL/hr) but begins to tail off (20 mL/hr). How will you manage her now?

ANSWERS

1. The patient is febrile and tachycardic—features that can suggest an infection. She has additional symptoms and signs that indicate that the infection could be in her urinary tract: dysuria and urinary frequency along with suprapubic tenderness. Her urine dipstick shows nitrites in the urine. Bacteria present in the urine can produce enzymes that convert urinary nitrates to nitrites that show up on the dipstick test. Elderly people, particularly females, are more prone to urinary tract infections and often present with confusion.

2. The patient is showing signs of sepsis, probably urosepsis. Current guidelines for managing sepsis advise that the following investigations and treatments be commenced within an hour of sepsis being identified (www.survivingsepsis.org):

🔎 INVESTIGATIONS

1. Take blood cultures.
2. Send blood tests, including a lactate level (an elevated lactate level is strongly associated with increased morbidity and mortality).
3. Measure urine output and consider siting a urinary catheter if necessary.

Treatments

1. Give oxygen to patients with evidence of hypoxia.

2. Commence intravenous fluids.

3. Commence broad-spectrum antibiotics, ideally after taking blood cultures, but this should not delay antibiotic therapy.

In addition to the aforementioned tests, the patient will need a urine sample to be sent to the laboratory for microscopy, culture, and sensitivities. She will be started on broad-spectrum antibiotics, but if a specific bacteria is grown and the antibiotic sensitivities became available, her antibiotics may be changed to a more targeted therapy. A chest x-ray should be performed to exclude other causes of infection.

3. The patient is haemodynamically unstable. She should be given a fluid challenge by administering a bolus of intravenous fluids. A typical regimen would be 500 mL Hartmann's solution/Ringer's lactate/0.9% saline given over 15–30 minutes. She should be monitored for signs of response to this, such as an increase in blood pressure, normalisation of her heart rate, or an improvement in urine output. Her care may need to be escalated to the critical care unit, where inotropic drugs can be given along with close monitoring of her fluid status via a central venous line to improve her heart rate and blood pressure. The patient's daughter should be informed that her mother is very unwell and may not survive. If the patient is well enough, her wishes regarding intubation and resuscitation should be discussed with her.

🔑 KEY POINTS

1. Urinary tract infections can often present with non-specific symptoms, such as confusion and general malaise, particularly in elderly patients.
2. Early treatment according to the Surviving Sepsis protocol is key to ensuring patients have the best chance of surviving a serious infection.

CASE 20: HEADACHE IN PREGNANCY

History

A 28-year-old woman who is 34 weeks pregnant presents to the emergency department complaining of a headache. She reports feeling increasingly nauseous and vomiting several times that day. She has also noticed some ankle swelling over the past week. This is her first pregnancy, and she has been well up until this point. The patient has no past medical history, takes no regular medications, and has no significant family history to her knowledge. She is an ex-smoker with a 5 pack-year history and does not drink alcohol.

Examination

The patient appears comfortable at rest. Her heart rate is 70 beats per minute, and her blood pressure is elevated at 160/90 mmHg. Her blood pressure was measured three times, with each reading taken 10 minutes apart, and there was no significant change in the result. Her heart sounds are normal, and her chest is clear. A full neurological examination is significant for 6 beats of clonus at both ankles. The symphysis-fundal height was 34 cm (normal for the gestation), and the presentation is cephalic. The foetal heart rate is 130/min. Her urine has been dipped and shows the presence of protein.

? | **QUESTIONS**

1. What condition could this pregnant woman be experiencing?
2. How should this patient be managed?

ANSWERS

1. In a pregnant woman, elevated blood pressure (>140/90 mmHg) or a rise in baseline systolic blood pressure of >20 mmHg and/or diastolic blood pressure of >10 mmHg, along with the presence of 300 mg protein in a 24-hour urine collection, should alert you to the possibility of pre-eclampsia. Sustained clonus (>5 beats) is one of the neurological signs that can be present in pre-eclampsia.

Pre-eclampsia is a potentially life-threatening condition that affects women who are at 20 or more weeks of gestation. There are many theories as to why women develop pre-eclampsia, including an immune-mediated endothelial dysfunction to the foetus and hypoxia of the placenta.

If pre-eclampsia is not managed, the condition can progress to eclampsia, with a high risk of seizures, cerebral haemorrhage, and adult respiratory distress syndrome.

2. The obstetrics team, with support from a maternal medicine team in some centres, will usually lead care in patients who are 20 or more weeks pregnant. The patient's blood pressure will need to be controlled to prevent seizures and intracerebral haemorrhage. Labetalol is a commonly used antihypertensive in these situations, as there is very little placental transfer to the foetus. An infusion of labetalol can be set up and titrated according to the patient's blood pressure. Magnesium sulphate is often also given to help prevent seizures.

Steroids should be given to promote foetal lung maturity in case early delivery is needed. If the condition continues to progress, delivery of the foetus will be necessary. Signs of pre-eclampsia typically settle within 48 hours of delivery.

🔑 KEY POINTS

1. Pre-eclampsia should be suspected in pregnant women in the second and third trimesters who present with hypertension and evidence of proteinuria on urine dipstick.
2. A labetalol infusion may be required to manage hypertension, and magnesium may need to be given to prevent seizures. Ultimately, if pre-eclampsia progresses, early delivery of the foetus may be necessary.

CASE 21: EPIGASTRIC PAIN AND VOMITING

History

A 55-year-old man has presented to the emergency department with abdominal pain and vomiting. He says that the pain came on gradually over the preceding day. The pain is dull and constant in nature and is located over the upper area of his abdomen, radiating through to his back. He has had multiple previous admissions to hospital, which were primarily related to alcohol excess. Apart from three to four admissions related to trauma, there is no significant past medical history. His mother has type 2 diabetes, but there is no other significant family history. He is divorced, lives alone in a flat, and is not currently working. He admits to drinking around 50 units of alcohol per week and has been drinking particularly heavily over the last fortnight. He smokes 20 cigarettes per day.

Examination

The patient appears agitated and is repeatedly asking for analgesia. His heart rate is 110 beats/min, and his blood pressure is 112/74 mmHg. His heart sounds are normal, and his chest is clear. His abdomen is soft with tenderness over his epigastrium and right upper quadrant. His bowel sounds are normal.

🔎 INVESTIGATIONS

Blood tests:	Result
White cells	19.4
Haemoglobin	131
Platelets	160
Sodium	142
Potassium	3.9
Urea	8.4
Creatinine	85
CRP	140
Amylase	320
Glucose	14.7

? QUESTIONS

1. What is the most likely cause of this man's abdominal pain and vomiting?
2. How would you confirm your diagnosis, and what treatment could you give?

ANSWERS

1. The man has features of acute pancreatitis. Pancreatitis classically presents with upper abdominal pain radiating though to the back and vomiting. The serum amylase level is typically elevated, and the patent may have signs of an inflammatory response, such as a fever and a high white cell count. Patients are often jaundiced.

   Numerous factors predispose a person to developing pancreatitis, but gallstones and alcohol misuse are the leading causes in the UK.

   Acute pancreatitis can be life threatening, with mortality rates of up to 10%.

2. The clinical features plus the elevated serum amylase level support a diagnosis of acute pancreatitis. The Glasgow-Imrie score should be calculated—this is a score based on clinical criteria that helps to determine the severity of acute pancreatitis.

   An abdominal ultrasound scan may show inflammation and oedema of the pancreas as well as the presence of gallstones and can exclude other forms of abdominal pathology if the diagnosis is in doubt; bowel gas may obscure views, however. A CT scan will also show inflammation of the pancreas and may provide better views of the pancreas than an ultrasound scan. It will also help to exclude other causes of acute abdominal pain.

   The patient will need analgesia for his abdominal pain; regular intravenous paracetamol should be commenced, but opioid medication is typically required. He should be kept 'nil by mouth', and intravenous fluids should be prescribed. Due to third-space losses (where fluid moves from the intravascular space to the interstitial space), aggressive fluid hydration may be required to maintain the patient's blood pressure. Although there is little supporting evidence for this, intravenous antibiotics are often given. A nasogastric tube may be sited to decompress the stomach and reduce the activity of the pancreas.

   As patients can develop an acute kidney injury or even acute respiratory distress syndrome, there should be a low threshold for involving the critical care team to assist with the patient's care. Blood tests should be performed at least daily to monitor the full blood count, renal function, liver function, and coagulation function. A blood gas sample should be obtained to monitor the lactate level, which can become elevated in sepsis or severe inflammation.

   As pancreatitis progresses, patients can develop hyperglycaemia due to impaired insulin production by the pancreas. In this case the patient's high blood glucose level may be related to the pancreatitis or possibly undiagnosed type 2 diabetes mellitus (note the family history). Hypocalcaemia may also become an issue, as the inflamed pancreas generates increased levels of free fatty acids that chelate calcium salts, which then precipitate in the abdominal cavity.

   In severe cases, surgical intervention may be needed to remove necrotic pancreatic tissue or to remove gallstones.

🔑 **KEY POINTS**

1. Pancreatitis usually presents with upper abdominal pain radiating though to the back and vomiting. Risk factors include gallstones and alcohol misuse.
2. Acute pancreatitis can be a life-threatening condition. Patients should be kept 'nil by mouth' with intravenous fluids and analgesia. Close monitoring of the patient's observations, clinical condition, and blood results will need to be carried out. Surgery may need to be performed.

CASE 22: FEVER IN A RETURNING TRAVELLER

History

A 29-year-old man presents to the emergency department complaining of a 2-day history of headache and vomiting. The headache is primarily frontal with retro-orbital pain. The patient does not report any associated neck stiffness or photophobia. He has vomited bilious matter four to five times over the past 2 days and has ongoing nausea but denies abdominal pain or diarrhoea. He has not measured his temperature during the illness, but has experienced several episodes of feeling cold and shivering uncontrollably. The patient additionally complains of generalised myalgia and pain in his hip and knee joints bilaterally. He has no significant past medical history and takes no regular medications. He denies recent unprotected sexual intercourse and has no unwell contacts. Earlier this week, he returned from a 3-week holiday with his family in the south of Kerala, India. He did not receive any immunisations or take antimalaria prophylaxis for this trip.

Examination

Observations: T 38.7°C, HR 108 bpm, BP 110/70 mmHg, RR 20, SpO$_2$ 99% on room air.

The patient is clearly in pain but looks otherwise well. There is an erythematous maculopapular rash over his trunk. There is no palpable cervical, axillary, or inguinal lymphadenopathy. His heart sounds are dual with no added murmurs and no stigmata of endocarditis. His chest is clear. His abdomen is soft and non-tender. Neurological examination is unremarkable. The patient does not have a positive Kernig's sign—there is no neck stiffness and no photophobia. There is no obvious joint swelling, but the patient's muscles are tender on palpation throughout.

🔍 INVESTIGATIONS

- Blood tests—WCC 2.9, Hb 148, Plt 105, Na 135, K 4.2, creat 73, bili 11, ALT 120, ALP 54, INR 1.2, and CRP 80
- Blood film—mild leucopenia and thrombocytopenia observed; thick and thin films performed—no evidence of malaria parasites
- Chest x-ray—clear lung fields
- CT brain—no intracranial pathology seen

❓ QUESTIONS

1. What is your differential diagnosis for this patient, and which tests would you perform in the acute setting?
2. A diagnosis of acute dengue fever is subsequently made. What features of this infection may develop over the coming days?
3. How will you treat this patient acutely, and what advice would you give him to prevent re-infection with the dengue virus in the future?

ANSWERS

1. This patient presents with headache, fever, myalgia, arthralgia, and rash, and his blood results show leucopenia, thrombocytopenia, and transaminitis. A number of acute infections can present with these features, including HIV in the seroconversion stage, as well as the hepatitis viruses. Common viruses, including Epstein-Barr virus (EBV) and cytomegalovirus (CMV), should also be considered, and serological tests should be performed for all of the aforementioned viruses.

   In view of the patient's headache, a diagnosis of meningitis (viral, bacterial, or fungal) should also be considered, although he does not have signs of neck stiffness or photophobia. Depending on how the patient progresses over the next few hours, empirical treatment followed by a diagnostic lumbar puncture may be indicated.

   He has recently returned from India, where infections such as dengue and chikungunya are prevalent. Although the risk of malaria infection is low in the region that this patient travelled to, this diagnosis should still be considered and a further two blood films should be sent to exclude malaria.

2. Dengue fever is an infection that is primarily transmitted by the female *Aedes aegypti* mosquito. Infected people are typically asymptomatic or have only mild flu-like symptoms, but around 5% of patients develop more serious complications. Symptoms develop within 2–14 days of exposure, and typical features include a fever, a headache (which is often located around the retro-orbital region), myalgia, and arthralgia, all of which were reported by this patient.

   A measles-like or petechial rash may be present. Patients may develop petechiae around pressure sites, including the upper arm if a blood pressure cuff has been inflated there. Blood results classically show leucopenia, thrombocytopenia, and transaminitis. The symptoms and signs of infection generally resolve over the subsequent days.

   In severe cases, increased vascular permeability results in disseminated intravascular coagulation and subsequent haemorrhagic and thrombotic sequelae. Multi-organ failure can develop, and patients may require critical care support.

3. The treatment for dengue virus is supportive, with the primary focus being on rehydration therapy (oral or intravenous). Many patients are safely managed at home if they are not vomiting, but patients with underlying medical problems or those with moderate-severe dengue infection may require inpatient care. Complications, including disseminated intravascular coagulation, encephalopathy, and haemodynamic instability, can develop. Intravenous fluids, blood products, and inotropic support are required in severe cases.

   Prevention of infection on an individual level involves avoiding insect bites by covering the skin, particularly in the evening; using mosquito nets at night; and utilising insect repellents. On a larger scale, the infection can be preventing by controlling habitats of the *A. aegypti* mosquito, which consist of bodies of open water.

   Infection with dengue virus may result in immunity to that individual subtype, but people will remain susceptible to other dengue subtypes. Newly developed vaccines have been introduced that have variable degrees of effectiveness in preventing infection with the dengue virus, and these may become more widely used in the coming years.

🔑 KEY POINTS

1. Patients infected with dengue virus are often asymptomatic or develop only mild, influenza-like symptoms. A small proportion of patients develop more severe features, including disseminated intravascular coagulation, encephalopathy, and haemodynamic instability.
2. Treatment of dengue virus is primarily supportive. People travelling to areas where dengue is endemic should take measures to prevent mosquito bites where possible.

CASE 23: SHORTNESS OF BREATH DURING A SICKLE CELL CRISIS

History

A 22-year-old man has been admitted to hospital with severe pain in his legs. He is known to have sickle cell disease and says that his pain is typical for his sickle crises. He was initially given opiate analgesia and intravenous fluids, and after 24 hours his pain had largely settled. He now complains of shortness of breath and right-sided chest pain. His past medical history is otherwise unremarkable, and his sickle cell disease has been generally very well-controlled over recent years. The patient takes regular penicillin V (prophylaxis against *Streptococcus pneumoniae* infections). He works as a laboratory assistant and does not drink alcohol or smoke cigarettes.

Examination

The patient appears dyspnoeic and distressed. He is afebrile. His heart sounds are normal, but his heart rate is 120 beats per minute. He has coarse crackles at both lung bases. His SpO_2 is 87% on room air. His abdomen is soft and non-tender. There is no peripheral oedema.

🔍 INVESTIGATIONS

- Arterial blood gas (taken on room air): pH 7.43, pCO_2 3.1, pO_2 7.4, lactate 2.7, BE +1, HCO_3 24

❓ QUESTIONS

1. How would you interpret the blood gas results?
2. What is the probable diagnosis?

DOI: 10.1201/9781003241171-23

ANSWERS

1. The arterial blood gas results demonstrate type 1 respiratory failure. The patient is hypoxic and is hyperventilating to try to improve his oxygenation. He is therefore blowing off more carbon dioxide, which is why the pCO_2 level is low.

2. The patient is likely experiencing a sickle cell chest crisis. When a patient is experiencing a sickle cell crisis, the misshapen sickle cells occlude the small blood vessels and cause hypoxia and tissue damage. When the sickle cells infiltrate the lungs, this can result in a sickle chest crisis.

   He will need urgent treatment with antibiotics and intravenous fluids. He should be given oxygen to increase his saturations to above 94%. A chest x-ray should be performed to look for signs of infection, infiltration, infarction, or fluid overload. He will need close observation and may need to be transferred to a high-dependency unit.

   If the crisis is not improving, the patient should be given a blood transfusion to introduce normal red cells to the circulation. Alternatively, if the haemoglobin level is too high to allow a transfusion to be carried out safely, an exchange transfusion may be carried out, whereby some of the patient's own blood is removed while donated blood is transfused.

   This condition can be life-threatening, and early involvement from senior medical doctors and possibly the critical care team may be necessary.

🔑 KEY POINTS

1. A chest crisis should be suspected in patients with known sickle cell disease who develop hypoxia.
2. A chest crisis can be fatal, so patients should be reviewed early for consideration of antibiotics, intravenous fluids, oxygen, and possibly a blood transfusion to try to improve the hypoxic tissue damage.

CASE 24: CHEST PAIN RADIATING TO THE BACK

History
A 74-year-old woman has presented to the emergency department with central chest pain radiating through to her back. This has lasted for 4 hours. She describes the pain as tearing in nature and scores it as 10/10 in severity. Her medical history is significant for hypertension, for which she takes regular indapamide tablets. She takes no other medications. The patient is a retired artist who lives with her husband and is independent for all activities of daily living. She has never smoked and does not regularly drink alcohol.

Examination
The patient is clearly uncomfortable, despite opiate analgesia being given immediately upon arrival. Her heart rate is 120 beats per minute. Her blood pressure is 102/50 mmHg in her left arm and 80/38 mmHg in her right arm. There is a loud, early diastolic murmur, which is loudest at the aortic region. There is a collapsing pulse. Her chest is clear. Her abdomen is soft and non-tender. There is no peripheral oedema. Figure 24.1 shows a chest x-ray.

🔍 INVESTIGATIONS

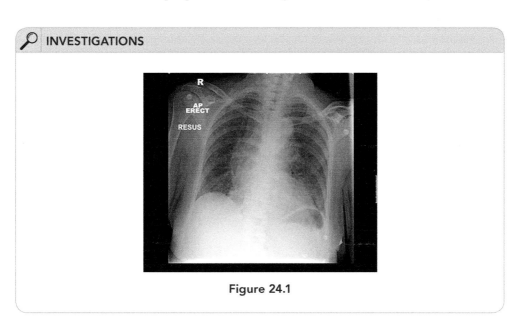

Figure 24.1

❓ QUESTIONS

1. What does the chest x-ray show?
2. What is the likely diagnosis?
3. How would you treat this woman?

DOI: 10.1201/9781003241171-24

ANSWERS

1. Tearing chest pain radiating to the back may indicate that the patient is experiencing an aortic dissection. This occurs when the inner lining of the aorta shears away from the vessel wall and blood flows between the layers, separating them. This can lead to aortic rupture, which has an 80% mortality rate.

   When the ascending thoracic aorta and/or the aortic arch is involved, this is referred to as a type A dissection, whereas type B dissections involve the descending thoracic aorta. The disparity in blood pressure between the arms indicates that the arch is involved.

   The chest x-ray shows a widened mediastinum. This can indicate that there is dissection of the thoracic aorta. The clinical signs of differing blood pressure in each arm, tachycardia, and aortic regurgitation (early diastolic murmur in the aortic region, collapsing pulse) are compatible with this diagnosis.

2. You should ensure that the patient has good intravenous access and that cross-matched blood is available for transfusion. Her blood pressure and heart rate will need to be closely monitored. To prevent further shearing of the aorta, the patient's systolic blood pressure will need to be kept below 100 mmHg. An infusion of a beta-blocker drug (e.g. labetalol), is typically used to do this.

3. The patient will need a central venous line and should be transferred either directly to theatre for an aortic repair or to a critical care unit for initial stabilisation. The critical care team, the anaesthetists, and surgeons should be notified about the patient immediately. Ultimately, the patient will need an aortic repair to be done as soon as possible.

🔑 KEY POINTS

1. Central chest pain radiating to the back should alert to the possibility of aortic dissection.
2. Early involvement of the surgical, anaesthetic, and intensive care teams will be needed to manage the patient, who is likely to need aggressive stabilisation and surgery.

CASE 25: SHORTNESS OF BREATH

History

An 80-year-old man has presented to the emergency department complaining of severe shortness of breath. He has been feeling increasingly dyspnoeic over the last fortnight and is now unable to walk short distances before becoming short of breath. He feels that his legs are becoming "too heavy to lift". He is also short of breath at night and has gone from sleeping with three pillows to sleeping upright in his chair. He complains of a cough productive of frothy pinkish sputum but has not experienced any fevers. He reports a history of hypertension and unspecified heart disease but has stopped taking his diuretic medication recently due to urinary frequency and occasional urinary incontinence. He lives alone and is normally independent for all activities of daily living. He is an ex-smoker with a 30 pack-year history and drinks alcohol occasionally at social events.

Examination

The patient is unable to speak in full sentences due to his dyspnoea. On auscultation of his chest, there are fine inspiratory crackles in the lower and mid zones bilaterally. His heart rate is 96 beats/min, and his blood pressure is 150/90 mmHg. A third heart sound is audible at the left sternal edge, but there are no audible murmurs. His jugular venous pressure (JVP) is raised at 8 cm. His abdomen is soft and non-tender. There is pitting oedema to the level of his knees.

🔍 INVESTIGATIONS

- An arterial blood gas shows hypoxia (type 1 respiratory failure).
- A chest x-ray (Figure 25.1) shows bilateral fluffy areas consistent with pulmonary infiltrates.

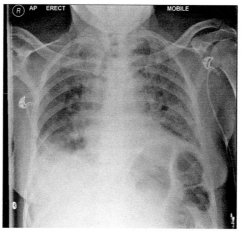

Figure 25.1

? QUESTIONS

1. Why has the patient become short of breath?
2. What would be the appropriate management?

DOI: 10.1201/9781003241171-25

ANSWERS

1. The patient has developed pulmonary oedema. He is known to have heart failure, but this has worsened over the past 2 weeks. He has stopped taking his diuretics because of the increased urinary output that resulted from the medication. This has led to fluid overload, as evidenced by signs including an elevated JVP, peripheral oedema, and fine crackles in the lungs indicative of pulmonary oedema.

2. The patient should be given oxygen via a face mask to improve his hypoxia and dyspnoea. His urine output will need to be measured accurately, ideally via passing urine into bottles, but a urinary catheter may need to be sited instead.

   A diuretic will need to be given to offload the fluid in the lungs. This can be with intravenous boluses of a diuretic, such as the loop diuretic furosemide. Alternatively, you can set up a continuous infusion of furosemide that can be titrated (increased or decreased accordingly) in line with the patient's blood pressure. Furosemide will cause a diuresis, where the kidneys excrete large volumes of fluid via the urine. The reduction in circulating fluid volume may lead to a reduction in blood pressure, so this should be monitored closely.

   Diuretics should be given intravenously initially, as the bowel can become oedematous in states of severe fluid overload, and gastrointestinal absorption is therefore reduced.

   Glyceryl trinitrate (GTN) can also be given as an infusion. GTN increases the availability of nitrous oxide and thus promotes vasodilatation and reduces both preload and afterload. If the patient is still uncomfortably dyspnoeic, a small dose of opiate analgesia, such as morphine, can be given to reduce the respiratory drive.

   For patients with hypotension who are unable to tolerate a furosemide or GTN infusion, or those who remain hypoxic despite the previous medical treatment, non-invasive ventilation (NIV) can be beneficial. NIV can redistribute fluid in the lungs and open up collapsed alveoli through positive pressure. This reduces the work of breathing and can improve the cardiovascular status by reducing the venous return and afterload. Patients with heart failure that have not responded to diuretic therapy should be considered for NIV in a critical care unit setting.

   The patient should have his fluid balance reviewed daily, with a clinical examination assessing his JVP and for the presence of pulmonary oedema and peripheral oedema. He should also be weighed daily and have his fluid input and output charted hourly. A 1–1.5 L fluid restriction may also be actioned for the initial days following his presentation. His electrolytes (sodium, potassium, magnesium) and creatinine levels should be monitored daily whilst he is receiving intravenous diuretics.

   Although this case of acute heart failure has likely been caused by the patient stopping his regular diuretic therapy, other causes, such as atrial fibrillation with a rapid ventricular rate or hyperthyroidism, should also be excluded.

🔑 **KEY POINTS**

1. Clinical signs of congestive cardiac failure include fine late inspiratory crackles in the lung bases, added heart sounds, an elevated JVP, and peripheral oedema.
2. Acute treatment usually consists of oxygen, intravenous furosemide, and catheterisation to monitor fluid balance. A small dose of morphine may be given to improve symptoms of dyspnoea.
3. For patients who do not improve with diuretics, NIV may be needed to redistribute fluid in the lungs.

CASE 26: RECURRENT ABDOMINAL PAIN

History

An 18-year-old woman attends the emergency department after developing severe abdominal pain. The pain came on gradually throughout the day, and she is now in too much pain to walk. She has been vomiting for the past few hours. She says that she has experienced recurrent episodes similar to this over the last 2–3 years, although they have typically been less severe and have resolved after a few hours. On direct questioning, she says that she thinks her cousin also suffers from similar intermittent episodes of abdominal pain. She has no other past medical history and takes no regular medications. She is currently studying at university, and prior to this, she had lived with her family in Cyprus, Greece. She drinks 15 units of alcohol per week and occasionally smokes cigarettes.

Examination

The patient is visibly uncomfortable. She is febrile (38.1°C). Her heart sounds are normal, and her chest is clear. Her abdomen is diffusely tender, and there are signs of guarding throughout but no rebound tenderness. She had an appendectomy scar in the right iliac fossa. The examination was otherwise unremarkable.

? QUESTIONS

1. What is the likely underlying diagnosis affecting this young woman and possibly her cousin also?
2. How would you manage this patient's condition?

DOI: 10.1201/9781003241171-26

ANSWERS

1. This lady gives a classic history of familial Mediterranean fever (FMF). Patients present with fevers and often have abdominal pain that mimics peritonitis on examination. Joint pains, pleuritis, and pericarditis are also common during flares of FMF.

   FMF is a condition that is inherited in an autosomal recessive pattern. A mutation in the *MEFV* gene is responsible.

2. The acute management of FMF is typically supportive. Intravenous fluids and simple analgesia usually suffice to help the patient feel better until the attack passes. Unfortunately, doctors often diagnose appendicitis during the first attack, and patients can go on to have an unnecessary appendicectomy.

   Colchicine, a drug usually given in gout and other rheumatological conditions, may be prescribed prophylactically to reduce the frequency of FMF attacks, although the mechanism of action for colchicine in this situation is uncertain. The drug is often poorly tolerated due to common side effects of abdominal discomfort and diarrhoea.

   FMF is suspected when there is a clear history of recurrent attacks with no obvious underlying cause, particularly if other family members have already received a diagnosis of FMF. If the diagnosis is in doubt, genetic studies can be carried out to identify mutated *MEFV* genes. Patients with FMF can go on to develop amyloidosis—a condition where abnormal proteins build up in the kidneys, heart, and lungs leading to disease.

KEY POINTS

1. FMF is an autosomal recessive disorder that typically affects people with a Mediterranean ethnic background. People present with recurrent episodes of inflammation, usually abdominal pain, but myositis, pericarditis, and pleuritis can also occur.
2. Patients with FMF are often given colchicine prophylactically to prevent flares of the condition. This drug also slows the progression to potentially developing amyloidosis.

History

A 52-year-old man has been referred by his family doctor to the respiratory outpatient clinic following several episodes of haemoptysis. He describes a 3- to 4-month history of a cough that is typically dry and has been present throughout the day and evening. Over recent days, he has experienced several episodes of haemoptysis, where he has expectorated an estimated 5 mL fresh blood on each occasion. He describes feeling fatigued and generally unwell over the past few months and has struggled to maintain his weight, unintentionally losing 8 kg in 12 weeks. He has been feeling feverish throughout the day but has not noticed that this is particularly worse at night. He has no unwell contacts and last travelled abroad to Nigeria 6 months earlier. His past medical history includes pulmonary tuberculosis, which was treated in Nigeria 4 years ago, although the patient is unsure if he completed the course of treatment. He takes no regular medications and has no known drug allergies. He works as a primary school teaching assistant and is married with two children. He has never smoked and does not drink alcohol regularly.

Examination

Observations: T 37.6°C, HR 90, BP 128/84, RR 16, SpO$_2$ 98% on room air

The patient is alert and orientated. Cardiovascular examination is unremarkable, and his chest is clear to auscultation. His abdomen is soft and non-tender. There is no peripheral oedema. There is no palpable cervical, axillary, or inguinal lymphadenopathy.

🔍 INVESTIGATIONS

- Chest x-ray: see Figure 27.1

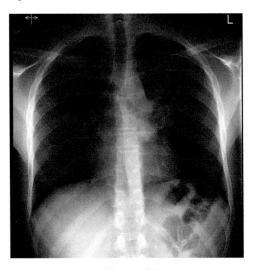

Figure 27.1

Sputum smear: positive for moderate numbers of acid-fast bacilli
Sputum culture: growth of *Mycobacterium tuberculosis*:

DOI: 10.1201/9781003241171-27

- Isoniazid—resistant
- Rifampicin—resistant
- Ethambutol—sensitive
- Pyrazinamide—sensitive

? QUESTIONS

1. What abnormalities are seen on this chest x-ray?
2. In light of the results, how should this patient be treated?

ANSWERS

1. There is increased soft tissue density at the left hilum with airspace shadowing. The appearances may represent a simple bacterial infection, but tuberculosis should also be considered, as should malignancy.

2. Initial treatment for pulmonary tuberculosis comprises two antibiotics (isoniazid and rifampicin) for 6 months, with additional pyrazinamide and ethambutol treatment for the first 2 months of the 6-month treatment period.

   In this case, the results of the sputum polymerase chain reaction (PCR) and culture results show that this patient has multi-drug-resistant tuberculosis. The patient may have developed this due to incomplete treatment of his initial tuberculosis infection, or he may have developed this multi-drug-resistant infection following person-to-person transmission, and his initial antimicrobial regimen may not have provided adequate cover to treat the infection.

   Multi-drug-resistant tuberculosis develops when the *M. tuberculosis* organism is resistant to both rifampicin and isoniazid, two of the more potent first-line antimicrobial agents. Although rare, this infection is now seen throughout the world. In some cases, patients may acquire 'extensively drug-resistant tuberculosis', where their *M. tuberculosis* infection is resistant to treatment with rifampicin, isoniazid, and at least two additional core anti-tuberculosis drugs. This results in less effective, more expensive antimicrobial agents being used to treat the infection. Multi- and extensively drug-resistant tuberculosis can be particularly serious in immunocompromised patients with more severe infections, such as those with HIV infection, where delivering appropriate antimicrobial treatment may become increasingly challenging.

   Patients with suspected or known infectious multi-drug-resistant tuberculosis (e.g. those with pulmonary tuberculosis and a productive cough) should be advised to self-isolate at home. Patients who require hospital admission should be isolated in a negative-pressure side room to prevent spread of the infection. Isolation precautions can typically be de-escalated within weeks, depending on adherence to therapy, resolution of cough, and results of further sputum analyses (to look for the ongoing presence of acid-fast bacilli). This patient should be advised to self-isolate at home and will now need to commence treatment with a combination of anti-tuberculosis drugs, as determined by a tuberculosis specialist.

🔑 KEY POINTS

1. Multi-drug-resistant tuberculosis develops when the *M. tuberculosis* organism is resistant to both rifampicin and isoniazid. The infection may develop following inappropriate or incomplete treatment of tuberculosis, or it can be contracted by person-to-person transmission.
2. Extensively drug-resistant tuberculosis develops when the *M. tuberculosis* organism demonstrates widespread antimicrobial resistance, meaning that more expensive, less potent antibiotics may be required. The condition is becoming increasingly difficult to treat.

CASE 28: BLOODY DIARRHOEA

History

A 25-year-old man has presented to the emergency department with abdominal pain, vomiting, and bloody diarrhoea. He attended a party the previous day, and several other attendees have since been taken ill with presumed food poisoning. He is too unwell to provide any further history.

Examination

The patient appears pale and shocked. His mucous membranes are dry, and he appears to be clinically dehydrated. His heart rate is 110 beats/min, and his blood pressure is 90/50 mmHg. His chest is clear. His abdomen is soft but generally tender throughout. Bowel sounds are active and have a normal pitch.

🔍 INVESTIGATIONS

Blood test	Result
White cells	18.0
Haemoglobin	80
Platelets	48
Sodium	149
Potassium	7.2
Urea	24.5
Creatinine	280
Blood film	Fragments of red cells, suggestive of haemolysis

❓ QUESTIONS

1. What abnormalities can be seen in the blood results?
2. In view of the clinical picture and the blood results, what is the probable diagnosis?
3. What would be the appropriate management?

ANSWERS

1. The full blood count shows a high white cell count, suggesting infection. The haemoglobin is low, and the blood film report states that there is evidence of haemolysis (abnormal breakdown of red cells). The platelet count is also low (thrombocytopaenia).

   The blood tests also show that the patient has impaired renal function. Although no baseline results are available, it is likely that the patient has an acute kidney injury. The elevated serum potassium level is particularly concerning, as this puts him at risk of developing cardiac arrhythmias.

2. The history of bloody diarrhoea preceding renal failure and blood tests showing a haemolytic anaemia and thrombocytopaenia support a diagnosis of haemolytic uraemic syndrome. Most cases are caused by infection with the *Escherichia coli*-0157 strain of bacteria. Patients usually develop symptoms of food poisoning with bloody diarrhoea. The infection can be life-threatening and has a high mortality rate of up to 10%. Other differential diagnoses of bloody diarrhoea include *Campylobacter* or *Shigella* gastroenteritis.

3. A patient with these features should immediately be referred to a high-dependency unit. He has an acute kidney injury and is severely hyperkalaemic.

   The first step is to manage his hyperkalaemia. He should be given calcium gluconate to stabilise his myocardium in the present of hyperkalaemia. Insulin should be given along with dextrose to drive the potassium back into the cells. Salbutamol nebulisers can also be given to promote potassium entry into cells.

   His urine output should be measured, and a urinary catheter should be inserted to facilitate this. The patient may need haemodialysis until his renal function improves. Antibiotics are generally avoided in haemolytic uraemic syndrome, as they can stimulate the release of further endotoxins, although this is decided on a case-by-case basis with involvement from the local infectious diseases team.

   Plasmapheresis (plasma exchange to remove immune complexes) may need to be performed until the platelet count normalises.

   As stated earlier, up to 10% of patients will die from the infection. A further 10% will develop end-stage renal failure requiring renal replacement therapy.

🔑 KEY POINTS

1. Haemolytic uraemic syndrome is a triad of haemolysis, thrombocytopaenia, and renal failure, often secondary to *E. coli*-0157 infection.
2. Patients with haemolytic uraemic syndrome are likely to require care in a high-dependency setting. Haemodialysis may be required along with plasmapheresis.

CASE 29: PROGRESSIVE DYSPHAGIA IN A PATIENT WITH KNOWN MALIGNANCY

History

An 88-year-old man, accompanied by his family, presents to hospital complaining of difficulty swallowing. He has experienced progressive dysphagia and odynophagia over recent months and is now struggling to swallow soft and pureed food. He has developed a fever and productive cough over the past week and feels short of breath on minimal exertion. He has a history of advanced oesophageal cancer, which was diagnosed 6 months earlier. The patient has previously been treated with combined chemoradiotherapy, oesophageal dilatation, and an intraluminal stent. The oncology team recently stated that there would be no potential for further active treatment at this stage. The patient and his family supported this decision. His past medical history also includes chronic obstructive pulmonary disease, hypertension, ischaemic heart disease, congestive cardiac failure with a predicted ejection fraction of 30%, and chronic kidney disease. The patient takes regular ramipril 10 mg OD, bisoprolol 7.5 mg OD, indapamide MR 1.5 mg OD, atorvastatin 40 mg ON, and calcium carbonate/cholecalciferol 1 tablet BD. He lives with his wife, son, and daughter-in-law, all of whom assist with his activities of daily living and his personal care. The patient is normally able to mobilise short distances around a room with a frame (approximately 10 metres). He is a retired accountant and is an ex-smoker with a 40 pack-year history. He previously consumed alcohol to excess but does not drink any alcohol at present.

Examination

Observations: T 37.4°C, HR 108 bpm, BP 90/66 mmHg, RR 28, SpO$_2$ 94% on room air.

The patient appears drowsy and mildly confused. He is cachectic with an estimated body mass index of 16. He feels cool peripherally and is tachycardic. There is pitting oedema to above his knees. On auscultation of his chest, there are crackles at the bases bilaterally, which extend up to the mid zone on the right side. His abdomen is soft and non-tender.

🔍 INVESTIGATIONS

- Blood results—WCC 15.4, Hb 102, Plt 568, Na 130, K 3.1, creat 150 (baseline 100), CRP 290
- Chest x-ray—consolidation throughout the right lower lobe

❓ QUESTIONS

1. How would you manage this patient acutely?
2. Should the patient deteriorate further, what additional treatment would be appropriate?

ANSWERS

1. This patient has a progressive oesophageal malignancy and now presents with worsening dysphagia and signs of a pneumonia, which may be secondary to aspiration of food. He should be prescribed a course of broad-spectrum antibiotics and some intravenous fluids. As he is unlikely to have received appropriate nutrition over recent weeks, additional electrolyte levels (calcium, phosphate, and magnesium) should be measured, as these may need to be replaced.

2. At this point, you should approach the patient, along with his family (if the patient consents to their involvement), and discuss what treatment options would be appropriate if he were to further deteriorate. For example, cardiopulmonary resuscitation is unlikely to be successful in view of the patient's frailty, poor baseline function, and multiple co-morbidities and is unlikely to be in his best interests. Similarly, intubation and ventilation may not be appropriate, as the patient does not have a clear, reversible problem, and the patient may agree that ward-based care would be more suitable. If the patient agrees that cardiopulmonary resuscitation should not be performed in the event of cardiac arrest, then this should be clearly documented and the relevant paperwork to support this completed. Although decisions relating to resuscitation and escalation of care are ultimately medical decisions, the patient and their relatives should be involved in these discussions wherever possible with an aim to reach a consensus.

   The palliative care team should be contacted to discuss whether any supportive interventions, such as further oesophageal stenting, are possible. If the patient does continue to deteriorate despite intravenous antibiotics and fluids, further discussions with the patient and his family should be undertaken to establish whether the patient would want ongoing end-of-life care to continue at home, in a hospice, or in the hospital. Subcutaneous injections of analgesia, anti-emetics, and sedation in case of anxiety, should be prescribed if needed, and if the patient requires multiple doses of these, then a syringe driver can be set up to ensure ongoing symptom control.

> ### 🔑 KEY POINTS
>
> 1. It is important to establish your patients' views on cardiopulmonary resuscitation and what their wishes would be regarding further treatment options in the event of deterioration, particularly where patients have a life-limiting condition.
> 2. The palliative care team can provide support in managing symptoms and arranging further care options outside the hospital for patients with terminal or, in certain cases, chronic illness.

CASE 30: PROGRESSIVE LOWER LIMB WEAKNESS

History

A 23-year-old man has presented to hospital complaining of numbness and weakness in his legs. He says that the symptoms began 2 days earlier, when he initially noticed tingling in his feet and weakness in the ankle joints. He reports that his legs are now feeling weak up to the level of his thighs, and he has fallen over several times. He describes his legs as feeling heavy and numb to touch. He denies any shortness of breath and feels otherwise well, although he says that he has recently recovered from an episode of food poisoning that lasted for several days. He currently has no symptoms of fever, nausea, vomiting, diarrhoea, or dysuria. He has no significant past medical history and takes no regular medications. He works as an accountant, does not drink alcohol regularly, and has never smoked.

Examination

The patient appears comfortable at rest. Cardiovascular, respiratory, and abdominal examinations are unremarkable. Upon examination of the neurological system, the patient has reduced sensation to both light touch and pin-prick from S1 up to the level of L2. There is reduced power throughout the lower limbs, which is worse distally. The knee and ankle reflexes are absent bilaterally. The upper limbs and cranial nerves show no abnormalities, although the patient reports that he has developed a sensation of 'pins and needles' or tingling throughout his hands.

? QUESTIONS

1. This patient presents with an ascending paralysis following an episode of food poisoning. What is the likely diagnosis?
2. What is the main concern regarding this patient's condition? How will you monitor the progression of his disease?
3. Can you think of any specific treatments for this illness?

ANSWERS

1. The patient is likely to have Guillain-Barré syndrome (GBS). This is an ascending paralysis that occurs secondary to an inflammatory demyelination of the peripheral nerves. The demyelination develops in response to an immune response to a foreign antigen. There is usually no demyelination present in the central nervous tissue (brain and spinal cord).

   In this case the patient has probably had an infection with *Campylobacter jejuni*, as evidenced by the episode of food poisoning. An autoimmune response is triggered, leading to GBS.

   Although GBS is normally diagnosed based on clinical features, several investigations may aid diagnosis. Nerve conduction studies and electromyography typically show abnormalities in keeping with demyelinating disease. Cerebrospinal fluid obtained from a lumbar puncture may show an elevated protein level (usually greater than 0.55 g/L), although this is not always present in the early stages of the disease.

2. The most concerning feature of GBS is that it can ascend to involve the respiratory muscles. This can lead to paralysis of the diaphragm muscles and subsequent respiratory arrest. Patients should be monitored closely for signs of respiratory distress, and bedside spirometry should be performed every 4 hours to record the vital capacity. Doctors should have a low threshold for intubating and ventilating patients with GBS, as diaphragmatic paralysis can occur rapidly over a few hours with catastrophic consequences.

3. GBS is an autoimmune condition, and the mainstay of treatment is to remove the circulating autoimmune complexes. Plasmapheresis (plasma exchange) can be performed in addition to the administration of intravenous immunoglobulins (IVIg). Supportive management with fluids and oxygen may be necessary.

   Physiotherapy is key to regaining function, and involvement from occupational therapists may aid progress. Most patients return to baseline function within 1–2 months.

🔑 **KEY POINTS**

1. GBS presents with an ascending paralysis that can spread to involve the diaphragm and cause respiratory arrest.
2. Treatment may include plasmapheresis and immunoglobulin administration, as well as general supportive measures.
3. Support from physiotherapists and occupational therapists will promote an early recovery to baseline function.

CASE 31: SEIZURE AND AGITATION

History

A 48-year-old man collapsed in the street with total loss of consciousness and jerking of his arms and legs for several minutes, according to statements from eyewitnesses. He was reportedly drowsy and disorientated for approximately 10 minutes afterwards and then regained full consciousness. The patient confirms that he had bitten his tongue and had also been incontinent of urine during the episode. He has been admitted to hospital for further monitoring. He denies having had seizures previously and reports being otherwise well recently. Specifically, he denies any recent trauma or head injury, as well as any headache, fevers, cough, shortness of breath, chest pain, diarrhoea, vomiting, or dysuria. He admits to typically drinking a 75-cL bottle of vodka (30 units) daily but has been trying to cut down recently and has not consumed any alcohol at all for the past 48 hours. He initially seemed alert and orientated on arriving to hospital but now that he has arrived to a ward, the nurses note that he has been increasingly agitated. When he is reviewed on the ward round a few hours later, he appears unwell and has vomited several times.

Examination

The patient is diaphoretic and appears very agitated. His heart sounds are normal, and his chest is clear. His abdomen is soft and non-tender and bowel sounds are active. He is hallucinating, describing insects covering the walls, and his hands are notably trembling.

Observations: Temperature 37.8 °C, HR 104 beats/min, blood pressure 158/96 mmHg, respiratory rate 28/min, SpO_2 100% on room air.

INVESTIGATIONS

Blood test	Result
White cells	6.0
Haemoglobin	14.8
Platelets	196
Sodium	138
Potassium	4.5
Urea	6.7
Creatinine	97
CRP	<5

A CT head scan performed in the emergency department was unremarkable.

? QUESTIONS

1. What is the most likely cause of this patient's seizure?
2. What worrying features does the patient display upon arrival to the ward?
3. Could the deterioration have been prevented?

DOI: 10.1201/9781003241171-31

ANSWERS

1. There are many potential reasons as to why this patient has had a seizure for the first time. We know from the patient's history that he has been misusing alcohol for some time. He drinks around 200 units of alcohol per week. The recommended maximum alcohol intake per week is around 21 units.

   The first thing to rule out is an intracerebral bleed and a subsequent seizure related to this. Alcohol misuse increases the risk of intracerebral bleeds, primarily because traumatic head injuries are more likely to occur when an individual is intoxicated. Additionally, sustained alcohol misuse can lead to deranged liver function and therefore reduced production of vitamin K, which is essential for normal blood clotting properties. A long history of excessive alcohol intake can lead to cerebral atrophy, so the fragile blood vessels between the meningeal layers have to traverse a longer distance and are therefore more prone to bleeding in the event of a head injury. The normal CT head scan in this case excludes a large intracerebral bleed. A subdural haematoma can take hours or days to develop, so this should always be considered in patients who have sustained a head injury.

   You should also consider that electrolyte abnormalities commonly develop in patients with a history of heavy alcohol use, particularly hyponatraemia, which can precipitate seizures. Long-term alcohol misuse can lead to impaired immune responses, so patients with a history of alcohol excess are at increased risk of infections that could precipitate a seizure, such as meningoencephalitis or an intracerebral abscess.

   Next consider that the patient could be withdrawing from alcohol. Seizures are a common way for patients with alcohol withdrawal to present. This patient reports that he has suddenly stopped drinking and has not consumed any alcohol for 48 hours. The timing of his presentation and the fluctuation in his consciousness make a seizure secondary to alcohol withdrawal likely.

2. The patient is displaying signs of autonomic dysfunction, with tachycardia, hypertension, and diaphoresis. This could all be related to the sudden withdrawal of alcohol. If not managed appropriately, the patient may develop delirium tremens, which can be life threatening. Patients with alcohol misuse are prone to other neuropsychiatric conditions, such as Wernicke's encephalopathy and Korsakoff's psychosis, due to a long-standing lack of thiamine (vitamin B_1).

3. Based on the history of alcohol excess, it should have been recognised that this patient was at high risk of developing an alcohol withdrawal syndrome so that he could be treated according to a withdrawal protocol. Most hospitals use one of the recognised alcohol withdrawal assessment scoring systems to objectively grade the severity of alcohol withdrawal that the patient is experiencing.

   For example, the Clinical Institute Withdrawal Assessment for Alcohol score, commonly abbreviated to CIWA or CIWA-Ar (revised version) score, is used to closely monitor for signs of withdrawal. This is both an objective and subjective score, assessing for agitation, tachycardia, and sweating, which are early features of alcohol withdrawal. Patients are usually given small doses of benzodiazepine as per the recommendation on their alcohol withdrawal score. They may require regular doses of benzodiazepines, which can then be gradually reduced over the course of several days. Patients who are at risk of alcohol withdrawal should be started on high doses of thiamine, initially given intravenously. This can help to prevent development of Wernicke's encephalopathy and Korsakoff's psychosis.

When he has recovered, the patient should be referred to alcohol support services if he wishes to continue to abstain from alcohol consumption in the future. Alcohol liaison teams can additionally support people with safely reducing their alcohol intake gradually in the community until they are successfully consuming little or no alcohol.

🔑 KEY POINTS

1. Patients withdrawing from alcohol have an increased risk of developing seizures.
2. Patients with a history of alcohol excess who are at risk of alcohol withdrawal should be monitored closely using a scoring system such as the CIWA-Ar score and may require small doses of benzodiazepines to control their symptoms.

CASE 32: SUBSTANCE MISUSE

History

A 24-year-old man has been admitted to hospital with agitation and confusion. His flatmate called an ambulance, as he was concerned that the patient was withdrawing from 'G', a recreational drug that the patient has been taking regularly. The patient typically uses the drug hourly in the daytime and every 3 hours at night but has not used any in the past 24 hours. He is usually fit and well.

Examination

The patient appears agitated and slightly diaphoretic. His heart sounds are normal, and his chest is clear. His abdomen is soft and non-tender. A full neurological examination cannot be carried out, as the man is too agitated to comply, but he is noted to be markedly tremulous. Observations: temperature 37.6 °C, HR 110 beats per minute, BP 138/84 mmHg, respiratory rate 20/min, SpO_2 99% on room air.

🔍 INVESTIGATIONS

Blood test	Result
White	cells 10.0
Haemoglobin	170
Platelets	300
Sodium	139
Potassium	4.8
Urea	6.8
Creatinine	90
CRP	8

❓ QUESTIONS

1. How will you manage this patient's initial withdrawal?
2. What management should be considered in the longer term?

DOI: 10.1201/9781003241171-32

ANSWER

1. γ-Hydroxybutyric acid (GHB) and its prodrug, γ-butyrolactone (GBL), both commonly referred to as 'G', are now among commonly used recreational drugs in UK clubs, particularly in gay clubs, as well as in 'chemsex', whereby intentional sex occurs under the influence of psychoactive drugs. They are central nervous system depressants that can have both euphoric and sedative effects and are highly addictive when used in high quantities. GHB/GBL users who consume large quantities of the drug regularly may require very frequent doses and rapidly start to withdraw within a few hours without GHB/GBL.

   Withdrawal from GHB/GBL can be life-threatening. It is often managed in a critical care setting and can last for up to 7–10 days. As with alcohol withdrawal, patients often require benzodiazepines, but sometimes in very high doses, so they must be monitored closely for respiratory depression. Baclofen, a drug that activates GABA-B receptors, may also be an effective therapeutic addition when managing GHB/GBL withdrawal symptoms. As people using high volumes of GBL/GHB can rapidly deteriorate, advice from the local toxicology team should be sought wherever possible, and the high-dependency team should be made aware of the patient.

2. Long-term support should be offered wherever possible to help patients continue to abstain from using drugs and alcohol. A number of addiction support groups are usually available in the community, and information about these should be provided to the patient before they are discharged home. Many hospitals have substance misuse teams that can support patients both in hospital and back in the community and provide information about accessing rehabilitation and detox facilities.

🔑 KEY POINTS

1. GHB/GBL are now among the leading recreational drugs used in certain areas of the UK.
2. Withdrawal from GHB/GBL can be life-threatening and begins after only a few hours of stopping the drug in people who use large quantities regularly.
3. Advice should be sought from the hospital critical care team and a toxicology team if available.

CASE 33: UNILATERAL LEG SWELLING

History

A 38-year-old man presents to the emergency department complaining of painful right leg swelling. The leg swelling and pain have developed gradually over the preceding 48 hours. The patient has no significant past medical history and no previous hospital admissions. He does not take any regular medications. He has a background of current intravenous drug use and injects heroin several times per day and occasionally smokes crack cocaine. He has been admitted for observation and treatment.

Examination

The patient is febrile (T 38.4 °C) and appears flushed. His heart sounds are normal, with no audible murmurs. His heart rate is 110 beats per minute, and his blood pressure is 120/80 mmHg. His chest is clear on auscultation, and his oxygen saturations are 99% on room air. His abdomen is soft and non-tender. There were numerous puncture wounds of various ages visible over his groins bilaterally and wounds consistent with 'skin popping' over his calves, shins, and feet. The lower part of his right calf was erythematous and warm to touch, with localised oedema. He was febrile and tachycardic.

Initial Treatment

Intravenous antibiotics are given. Although the patient seems to improve initially, he later develops severe pain around the site of swelling and increased erythema. The pain is severe and seems out of proportion to the appearance of the leg swelling. He becomes progressively more unwell over the next day, with fevers, tachycardia, and hypotension.

? QUESTIONS

1. What differential diagnoses should you consider for the swollen leg at the time of his initial presentation?
2. What would be the appropriate management for his painful, swollen leg?
3. What is a likely cause of the deterioration with severe leg pain?

DOI: 10.1201/9781003241171-33

ANSWERS

1. This patient has swelling and erythema of his leg, which is also warm to touch. These signs point towards a diagnosis of cellulitis. Intravenous drug use increases the risk of cellulitis developing, as injection sites become infected, particularly if non-sterile needles and syringes are used and shared. Infection is also more likely when the patient's nutritional intake is poor. Repeated injection into the femoral veins can lead to the development of abscesses and sinus tract formation, and the groins should be examined to ensure that these are not present.

   A deep vein thrombosis should also be considered. Repeated venous puncture and low-grade infection promotes endothelial dysfunction and higher levels of clotting factors, all leading to increased risk of embolus formation.

2. The examination findings should often suggest whether an infection or a deep vein thrombosis is present. In this case, the patient is more likely to have cellulitis. Blood tests will probably show raised inflammatory markers. A swab of the infected tissue should be taken, as well as blood cultures if the patient is febrile, to attempt to identify a specific bacteria causing the infection. In the meantime, a course of broad-spectrum antibiotics should be commenced. If signs of sepsis are present (fever, tachycardia, hypotension), then intravenous fluids may need to be given, and the high-dependency team may need to be notified about the patient in case of deterioration. If a deep vein thrombosis remains high on the list of differential diagnoses, a Doppler ultrasound scan of the affected limb can also be arranged to assess for the presence of a venous thrombus.

3. Severe pain, out of proportion to an area of infection, should always alert you to the possibility of necrotising fasciitis. This is an infection caused by multiple bacteria, including group A streptococcus and methicillin-resistant *Staphylococcus aureus* (MRSA), that spread through the subcutaneous and deep tissues, releasing toxins that can lead to overwhelming sepsis. Patients with necrotising fasciitis often require admission to a high-dependency unit, and wounds may need to be debrided.

🔑 KEY POINTS

1. Unilateral leg swelling in a patient with intravenous drug use should prompt consideration of cellulitis or a deep vein thrombosis as possible diagnoses.
2. Necrotising fasciitis should be suspected in patients with severe, seemingly disproportionate pain. As pain is very subjective, the diagnosis can be hard to make. Early involvement of the surgical teams will allow debridement of the wound (if necessary) and improve morbidity.

CASE 34: VOMITING CAUSED BY NOROVIRUS

History

A 92-year-old woman is admitted with diarrhoea and vomiting. She reports having vomited more than 20 times over the preceding 48 hours and is now unable to tolerate any oral intake. She lives with her family, who have become increasingly concerned that she is becoming dehydrated. Other members of the family have experienced similar symptoms over the last week. Her past medical history includes hypertension and diet-controlled type 2 diabetes mellitus. Her drug history includes ramipril 2.5 mg OD and bendroflumethiazide 2.5 mg OD. She does not drink alcohol and has never smoked.

Examination

The patient has dry mucous membranes and looks fatigued. Her jugular venous pulse is not visible. Her heart sounds are normal, and her chest is clear. Her abdomen is soft with mild, generalised tenderness. Observations: temperature 37.3 °C, HR 98 beats/min, BP 84/40 mmHg, respiratory rate 24/min, SpO_2 98% on room air.

 INVESTIGATIONS

- Vomitus samples—positive for norovirus.

Initial Treatment

The patient is admitted for intravenous fluid hydration and initially appears to have made a good improvement. On the third day, she develops shortness of breath and a cough productive of green sputum. On auscultation, there are coarse crackles at the left lung base.

? **QUESTIONS**

1. How would you treat the patient's gastroenteritis?
2. Why may she have developed a chest infection?

DOI: 10.1201/9781003241171-34

ANSWERS

1. Norovirus, otherwise known as the winter vomiting bug, is an RNA virus that is a common cause of gastroenteritis. Typical symptoms include vomiting, diarrhoea, and abdominal pain. The virus is spread via the faecal-oral route, but can be airborne and so spreads rapidly among contacts. The virus is usually self-limiting, and symptoms usually resolve over several days.

   Oral rehydration solutions can be useful in treatment. Patients, usually the very young and the elderly, may become severely dehydrated with viral gastroenteritis. The patient in our clinical scenario has features of dehydration, with dry mucous membranes and a JVP that is hard to visualise. She also has tachycardia and is hypotensive, again suggesting that the patient is volume deplete. Hypotension and tachycardia are features of moderate-to-severe dehydration. She needs to be admitted for intravenous fluids and monitoring of her blood pressure and heart rate as a guide to her fluid status.

   Patients with diarrhoea and vomiting can also develop an acute kidney injury secondary to renal hypoperfusion, and the patient's renal function should therefore be monitored by measuring her serum creatinine concentration. Depending on the patient's blood pressure and renal function, it may be prudent to withhold her regular angiotensin-converting enzyme (ACE) inhibitor and diuretic. Ask the nursing team to record the patient's fluid status via an hourly chart to monitor her fluid input and output. Lastly, electrolyte abnormalities are common with severe gastroenteritis, and thus the patient's sodium, potassium, magnesium, and phosphate levels should be regularly checked whilst her symptoms persist.

2. The patient has developed signs of a lower respiratory tract infection, which could be secondary to an organism acquired either in the community or in the hospital. A community-acquired lower respiratory tract infection is diagnosed when symptoms begin in the community or within 48–72 hours of hospital admission. When symptoms develop after 48–72 hours in hospital, it is more likely that a patient has acquired an infection from the unit, and this is termed a hospital-acquired pneumonia. It is important to differentiate between the two, as hospital-acquired infections are more likely to be resistant to antibiotics.

   In patients who are vomiting and develop signs of a lower respiratory tract infection, an aspiration pneumonia should be considered. This occurs when small amounts of a foreign material, such as food, liquid, or vomit, enters the airway. This can cause a very serious, life-threatening pneumonia, and intravenous antibiotics should be started immediately. A chest x-ray may show signs of early inflammation in the lungs secondary to aspirated material.

   If there are concerns about the patient's ability to swallow safely, they should not eat or drink until a formal swallowing assessment has been carried out. Intravenous fluids should be commenced for patients with a potentially unsafe swallow until this assessment has been conducted. If a patient is considered to be at risk of ongoing aspiration, measures such as inserting a nasogastric tube may be appropriate.

CASE 42: ECCHYMOSIS

History

A 31-year-old woman has presented to the emergency department with significant bruising on her arms and legs that has been getting worse. She first noticed them 5 days ago when they started off as small bruises. She did not report any trauma to her limbs. She intended to visit her general practitioner (GP), but noticed they were now larger and more widespread. She has had no fevers, arthralgia, or recent viral infections, and she is not taking any medications. She has not travelled outside the UK in the last 5 years.

Examination

This woman looks systemically well. There is a marked petechial rash over her legs with large bruising on the arms and legs but no evidence of mucosal involvement. A cardiovascular and respiratory exam is normal. On abdominal examination there is no hepatosplenomegaly and there is no lymphadenopathy. Observations: temperature 36.8°C, heart rate 78 beats/min, blood pressure 135/67 mmHg, respiratory rate 18/min, SpO$_2$ 98% on room air.

🔍 INVESTIGATIONS

		Normal range
White cells	6.0	
Haemoglobin	11.1	
Platelets	15	
Sodium	133	
Potassium	3.7	
Urea	5.4	
Creatinine	65	
INR	1.0	
APTT	23	
Bilirubin	10	
ALT	12	
ALP	65	
Albumin	42	
CRP	3	
Blood film	Reduced platelet count, no abnormal white cells	

❓ QUESTIONS

1. What is the most likely diagnosis?
2. How should this patient be managed?

ANSWERS

The main abnormality in the results is the very low platelet count. The most likely diagnosis is immune thrombocytopenia (ITP), but this requires exclusion of other causes of thrombocytopenia and to screen for secondary causes of ITP. Of note, the blood film did not show evidence of haematological malignancies or fragmented red cells (schistocytes), and there is no clinical evidence of sepsis. The rhesus status and direct antiglobulin test also forms part of the primary evaluation. Other secondary causes of ITP include IgA deficiency, common variable immunodeficiency, HIV, hepatitis C, and in some regions of the world (Southern and Eastern Europe, South America, and Asia) *Helicobacter pylori*. Thyroid function test is required, as hypothyroidism and hyperthyroidism can lead to mild thrombocytopenia, which is reversible on restoration of euthyroid status. Additionally, hyperthyroidism may develop in the long term in up to 14% of ITP patients due to thyroglobulin antibodies development. Hepatitis B and pregnancy tests should be carried out, as treatment of ITP may require transfusion and/or immunosuppressive drugs. An abdominal ultrasound should be performed to check the size of the spleen and look for any other masses, as an enlarged spleen indicates an alternative diagnosis. Bone marrow aspirate and biopsy are only considered in the context of abnormal blood film or cases that are refractory to treatment. In the absence of medications (e.g. quinine, rifampicin, co-trimoxazole, heparin) and infective causes, ITP is the likely cause.

A platelet count of 30×10^9/L is generally considered a threshold for treatment due to the increased risk of bleeding once platelet count is below this level. However, this threshold should consider age, lifestyle factors, and co-morbidities that may predispose to bleeding. As the patient's bruising is worsening, she should be treated with prednisolone and/or intravenous immunoglobulin. These treatments take 1–5 days to have a clinical effect. There is increasing body evidence to support anti-D immunoglobulin as an alternative or adjunct in those adult ITP patients who are rhesus-positive and non-splenectomised. If there is life-threatening bleeding, such as an intracranial bleed, platelet transfusion in addition to immunoglobulin/steroid therapy can be given, but the duration of action is short-lived and may need to be repeated. Tranexamic acid can also be administered, as this helps to inhibit fibrinolysis and stabilise clot formation, but this is contraindicated in the presence of haematuria, as it may precipitate renal tract obstruction. Spontaneous remission occurs in up to 10% of adult-onset ITP. Second-line medical therapies for adult patients with ITP who do not have an initial response to glucocorticoids or who have recurrent decreases in platelet counts after glucocorticoids are discontinued ($<50 \times 10^9$/L) include thrombopoietin receptor agonists (e.g. eltrombopag, romiplostim) and immunomodulators (e.g. rituximab), and they are used under specialist supervision. If bleeding episodes are poorly controlled despite first- and second-line medical therapy, a splenectomy can be considered, usually 12 months after the initial diagnosis.

? KEY POINTS

1. ITP is a diagnosis of exclusion, and there is no confirmatory test for it.
2. If the spleen is enlarged, then another cause is more likely, such as systemic lupus erythematosus (SLE).

CASE 43: PETECHIAE AND LIMB WEAKNESS

History

A 49-year-old woman suddenly developed right arm and leg weakness and has been brought to the emergency department. She describes a 1-week history of feeling tired, weak, and muddled. Her medical history includes hypertension and hypothyroidism. She is taking irbesartan and levothyroxine. She does not smoke and drinks wine only occasionally.

Examination

This woman has extensive petechiae over her legs. Cardiovascular, respiratory, and abdominal exams are normal. Neurological exam shows a right-sided mild hemiparesis with no sensation disturbance or visual disturbance. No higher cortical dysfunction is found. A CT head scan does not show any bleeding. Observations: temperature 37.8°C, heart rate 76 beats/min, blood pressure 150/89 mmHg, respiratory rate 16/min, SpO_2 96% on room air.

🔍 **INVESTIGATIONS**

		Normal range
White cells	9.0	
Haemoglobin	8.6	
Reticulocytes	5%	
Platelets	12	
Sodium	140	
Potassium	5.1	
Urea	16.2	
Creatinine	155	
INR	1.0	
APTT	35 seconds	
Blood film	Schistocytes and low platelet count	
Direct Coombs test	Negative	

❓ **QUESTIONS**

1. What is the most likely diagnosis?
2. How would you manage this patient?

DOI: 10.1201/9781003241171-43

ANSWERS

This patient has anaemia, thrombocytopenia, red cell fragments on blood film, normal clotting profile with petechiae, fever, neurological signs, and impaired renal function. These findings are consistent with thrombotic thrombocytopenic purpura (TTP). The classic description is a pentad of microangiopathic haemolytic anaemia (MAHA), thrombocytopenic purpura, neurological dysfunction, renal dysfunction, and fever. However, most cases of TTP do not have all five features, with up to 35% of patients not having neurological signs. The negative direct Coombs and coagulation tests are useful in differentiating from autoimmune haemolytic anaemia and disseminated intravascular coagulation, which are important differential diagnoses of thrombocytopenia and MAHA. Others include haemolytic uraemic syndrome (HUS) associated with *Escherichia coli* 0157:H7 infection, malignant hypertension, autoimmune diseases including vasculitis, viral infections (cytomegalovirus, adenovirus, herpes simplex), severe bacterial infections (pneumococcal and meningococcal infections), underlying malignancies, severe pancreatitis, and cancer-associated thrombotic microangiopathy.

TTP is caused by an autoimmune-induced deficiency of the enzyme ADAMTS-13 that cleaves ultra-large von Willebrand factor (vWF) multimers released from the vascular endothelium. An accumulation of large vWF forms platelet aggregates that cause microvascular thrombosis in organs such as the brain, heart, and kidneys. At presentation, the typical platelet count is $10–30 \times 10^9$/L and the haemoglobin level is usually 80–100 g/L. The lactate dehydrogenate (LDH) level is elevated due to haemolysis and tissue ischaemia. The reduction in haptoglobin level and reticulocytosis also confirms haemolysis. Troponin is elevated in 50% of cases reflecting cardiac involvement, and coronary artery obstruction is a common fatal complication. ADAMTS-13 assay (activity levels and antibody testing) should be sent immediately. Other baseline tests that are important include (i) calcium, which may reduce during plasma exchange; (ii) pregnancy test in women of childbearing age; and (iii) viral serology, including hepatitis A, B, and C and HIV, to exclude as underlying cause of TTP and for pre-blood product administration purposes.

Untreated TTP is fatal, and the patient presents with neurological and renal dysfunction. Immediate management should be to arrange plasma exchange within 24 hours of presentation in a high-dependency area. She should also be started on immunosuppression (e.g. intravenous methylprednisolone and rituximab) and caplacizumab, an inhibitor of ultra-large vWF and platelet interactions. The duration of plasma exchange can be gauged by clinical improvement and a rise in platelet count and ADAMTS-13 level. Platelet transfusion should be avoided unless there is severe active bleeding. Drugs that may trigger TTP should be avoided (e.g. calcineurin inhibitors, ticlopidine, clopidogrel, quinine, and statins).

? KEY POINTS

1. Plasma exchange, immunosuppression, and caplacizumab are the main treatments in the acute presentation of TTP.
2. TTP presents with neurological signs in about half of cases.
3. The pathophysiology is similar to HUS. Severe ADAMTS-13 deficiency (<5%) has a 90% specificity in distinguishing TTP from HUS. Please refer to Case 28.

History

A 37-year-old woman attended the emergency department with difficulty breathing and a wheeze. Symptoms started a couple of days ago. She was well prior to presentation and does not tend to have episodes like this for several years. She tried her blue inhaler that she's had for a long time, but it wasn't working. Her children were recently unwell with mild coryzal symptoms. She used to have childhood hay fever but grew out of it. She has a history of mild asthma but generally did not need her inhalers. She does not smoke.

On observation the patient was breathlessness but coherent and able to talk in complete sentences. On examination her temperature was 37.2°C, pulse rate was 95 bpm, blood pressure was 115/75 mmHg, respiratory rate 22/min, and oxygen saturations 93% on room air. A peak flow was attempted, and the best one obtained was 320 L/min. The patient can't recall having performed a peak flow for a long time, but her best predicted peak flow is estimated to be 440 L/min. On examination she had a wheeze bilaterally and symmetrical chest expansion. No other abnormalities were found on examination. A blood gas was performed, and her paO_2 was 10 kPa on room air, with a $paCO_2$ of 4.0 kPa. Chest x-ray (CXR) showed no evidence of pneumonia or pneumothorax. A blood test showed elevated eosinophils of 0.75×10^9/L.

? **QUESTIONS**

1. What is the most likely presenting diagnosis in this situation?
2. How is this condition diagnosed?
3. What would be the most appropriate management?

ANSWERS

1. The diagnosis here is an acute exacerbation of asthma. The patient presents with a recent onset of symptoms having been well a few days before. Her history does not suggest a history of poorly controlled asthma. In this case a trigger may have been a viral illness picked up from her children. The common cold is a well-known trigger (e.g. rhinoviruses, respiratory syncytial virus [RSV], enteroviruses, coronaviruses). Other triggers could include exercise, cold weather, pollen, or other allergens including occupational exposure and particulates in air pollution, and this should be enquired about in the history.

   Asthma is characterised by any of the symptoms of breathlessness, wheeze, cough, and chest tightness that are episodic in nature and accompanied by objective assessment of expiratory airflow limitation.

   It is likely she has allergic asthma, as she has a history of asthma diagnosed in childhood accompanied by a history of hay fever, another allergic condition. Another consideration is non-allergic asthma, which is diagnosed in adults who do not have a history of childhood-onset asthma or allergic conditions.

2. Diagnosis is based on objective tests for airway flow limitation or evidence of airway inflammation. This can also be supported by a clinical history of typical symptoms looking for triggers, episodic nature, and history of allergies or family history of asthma and allergies. Fractional exhaled nitric oxide (FeNO) is used to detect the degree of eosinophilic airway inflammation in asthma and can be used to support a diagnosis of asthma, as well as to guide disease control.

3. Immediate management in this case involves assessing the severity of an acute exacerbation of asthma based on the patient's ability to complete sentences, as well as heart rate, respiratory rate, oxygen saturations, peak flow recordings, and blood gas results. She is experiencing a mild to moderate episode, but this can quickly worsen to severe or life-threatening. In the current situation, supplementary oxygen should be given to maintain saturations in the 93%–95% saturation range. A high-dose, short-acting beta-2 agonist is given via an oxygen-driven nebuliser to relax the bronchial smooth muscle and inhibit bronchoconstrictor mediators from being released. A steroid is also administered either orally or parenterally if it cannot be taken orally. Steroids suppress inflammation and reduce the infiltration of eosinophils. Clinical response should be monitored regularly and a peak flow repeated to see improvement.

   Longer-term therapy will include controlling airway inflammation with inhaled corticosteroids and avoiding triggers if possible. Other treatments include leukotriene receptor antagonists, and in some patients difficult-to-treat asthma can be treated with biological therapies (e.g. anti-IgE monoclonal antibodies, anti-IL5 antibodies).

? KEY POINTS

1. An asthma diagnosis is based on an episodic cluster of symptoms with objective assessment of airflow limitation and/or airway inflammation.
2. The management of acute asthma depends on clinical indicators of mild, moderate, severe, or life-threatening features based on GCS, blood gas findings, peak flow, HR, RR, and oxygen saturations. PCO_2 levels should be lower than the normal range, as the patient's ventilatory rate is increased. If rising into the normal range, this could represent reduced ventilation and indicate worsening asthma.

CASE 45: DYSPHAGIA AND SHALLOW BREATHING

History

A 32-year-old woman has presented to the emergency department with increasing difficulty in swallowing and difficulty in breathing. She is also unable to lift her arms, and her head keeps drooping. These symptoms appeared after a recent chest infection. Last year she had visited her general practitioner (GP) because of double vision that worsened with reading and with intermittent weakness. She also noted difficulty in talking after prolonged speech. However, symptoms were mild and occasional only and no treatment was required. She has no medical history, is not on medications, and is generally fit and well.

Examination

This woman looks fatigued and has droopy eyelids. She breathes quickly and shallowly. A neurological examination reveals proximal muscle weakness and bilateral mild ptosis but no muscle wasting or abnormal reflexes. The rest of the cardiovascular, respiratory, and abdominal examination is unremarkable. Observations: blood pressure 127/62 mmHg, heart rate 62 beats/min, respiratory rate 28/min.

? QUESTIONS

1. What is the most likely diagnosis?
2. How would you manage this patient?

DOI: 10.1201/9781003241171-45

ANSWERS

This woman has dysphagia, respiratory distress, and generalised weakness. In the context of earlier intermittent symptoms of fatigue-induced muscular weakness affecting speech and vision, she is likely to suffer from myasthenia gravis (MG) and now presents in a myasthenic crisis. A crisis is often provoked within the first 2 years of diagnosis and is precipitated by infections, aspiration, or drugs.

MG is a chronic autoimmune disorder affecting the neuromuscular junction of skeletal muscles. Antibodies against the nicotinic acetylcholine receptor cause destruction of the post-synaptic membrane. Hence skeletal muscle weakness occurs. MG can affect just the ocular muscles or also can involve other muscle groups such as limb and axial muscles or oropharyngeal and respiratory muscles. Muscle weakness can be graded as mild to severe. Severe muscle weakness of the oropharyngeal and respiratory groups can compromise the airway. Infection can worsen MG.

Tests to confirm MG include serum anti-acetylcholine receptor antibody; if this is negative, anti-muscle tyrosine kinase antibody is commonly present. If antibodies are negative, repetitive nerve testing can be performed to demonstrate a successive decrement in action potentials. A CT chest is performed in newly diagnosed cases to rule out an associated thymoma. The major differential is Lambert-Eaton myasthenic syndrome (LEMS); however, in this case the history points towards MG and there are no autonomic features. LEMS is also usually associated with an underlying malignancy or with anti–voltage gated calcium channel (VGCC) antibodies in those without cancer. Other myopathies can present with muscle weakness, but they are not fatigue-induced—which is characteristic of MG.

This woman has a myasthenic crisis precipitated by pneumonia and is at risk of respiratory failure. Her forced vital capacity (FVC) should be measured: an FVC of 15 mL/kg or less would suggest the need for mechanical ventilator support. To reverse the process, she will need either intravenous immunoglobulin or plasma exchange. Even if she does not require intubation, she should be closely monitored by serial FVC and treated in an intensive care setting where intubation can be performed.

Once she has responded to acute treatment, pyridostigmine is required in the long term. Some patients with severe MG require regular intermittent intravenous immunoglobulin therapy every month. Other immunosuppressant therapy (e.g. prednisolone, azathioprine, ciclosporin) may be needed for maintenance treatment.

? KEY POINTS

1. Myasthenia crisis can be precipitated by infection, aspiration, trauma, drugs, surgery, or pregnancy.
2. MG presenting with oropharyngeal weakness or shortness of breath should alert you to potential respiratory compromise.

CASE 46: PAINFUL ANKLES AND RASH

History

A 40-year-old woman was referred by her general practitioner to ambulatory care with a 3-day history of multiple painful red nodules over the anterior aspect of her shins bilaterally. This was preceded by bilateral ankle pain and oedema in the last 2 weeks. There were no other mucosal manifestations of note. On system review, she did not have any cough, shortness of breath, change in bowel habits, night sweat, weight loss, or fever. She does not smoke and only drinks alcohol very occasionally. She has no previous past medical history and does not use any regular medications, including oral contraceptive pills There is no family or travel history of note.

Examination

There are multiple erythematous nodules over both shins that are 5–10 cm in size and very tender to touch. There is bilateral, non-pitting, ankle oedema that is tender to palpate. The rest of the examinations were unremarkable. Observations: temperature 37.5°C, heart rate 88 beats/min, blood pressure 100/70 mmHg, SpO$_2$ 100% on room air.

🔍 INVESTIGATIONS

White cells	7.0
Haemoglobin	11.2
Platelets	182
Sodium	135
Potassium	3.7
Urea	5.0
Creatinine	67
AST	12
ALT	18
ALP	78
Albumin	36
Corrected calcium	2.15
CRP	60
NT-pro BNP	<400 pg/mL
Urine beta-HCG	negative
Plain chest radiograph	bilateral hilar lymphadenopathy, no other changes

---

❓ QUESTIONS

1. What is the diagnosis?
2. How should this patient be managed?

DOI: 10.1201/9781003241171-46

ANSWERS

The tender erythematous nodules located on the front of both shins are erythema nodosum. This, together with ankle arthritis and bilateral hilar lymphadenopathy on chest x-ray, are features that are consistent with acute sarcoidosis or Löfgren's syndrome.

The most important differential diagnoses for bilateral hilar lymphadenopathy and erythema nodosum are tuberculosis, haematological malignancies, and sarcoidosis. Careful clinical assessments should be carried out for tuberculosis, the presence of 'B' symptoms, and chronic occupational exposure to dust for berylliosis and silicosis.

In a typical presentation, as in this case, a CT chest is not always necessary, but repeat chest x-ray within 3 months is recommended to look for interval changes. CT chest is helpful in characterising the lymphadenopathies and detecting parenchymal features that may not be evident on chest x-ray alone. It is also useful when the presentation is atypical to look for features that may point to other diagnoses. Definitive diagnosis of sarcoidosis can only be established by tissue biopsy, and this is considered when there is diagnostic uncertainty. It would not be necessary in this case. Full recovery for Löfgren's syndrome within 2 years is expected in most cases. Erythema nodosum and ankle arthritis should be managed by non-steroidal anti-inflammatory drugs (NSAIDs). Systemic immunosuppression is rarely necessary in Löfgren's syndrome. It is reserved for those that progress into a more severe form of lung disease or when other organs are affected. In this instance, oral corticosteroids are the first-line treatment.

Sarcoidosis is a multisystem disorder characterised by non-caseating granuloma. Therefore, it is prudent to look for extrapulmonary manifestations and to assess for target organ damage. This includes blood tests for liver function calcium and lung function test and 12-lead ECG. If shortness of breath is out of proportion to lung function test results, then echocardiogram should be considered to look for cardiac manifestations and pulmonary hypertension. Uveitis, cutaneous sarcoidosis, and rarely neurosarcoidosis can also occur. Raised serum angiotensin-converting enzyme (ACE) is sometimes seen in sarcoidosis but is not always the case. In those with raised serum ACE level, it may be useful as a marker for disease activity.

> **? KEY POINTS**
>
> 1. Acute sarcoidosis/Löfgren's syndrome is characterised by erythema nodosum, bilateral hilar lymphadenopathy, and ankle arthritis, and it usually resolves spontaneously.
> 2. It is important to conduct careful clinical assessment to rule out tuberculosis and haematological malignancies.

CASE 47: COLLAPSE ASSOCIATED WITH A HEADACHE

History

A 56-year-old woman has presented to the emergency department after collapsing at work. She was sitting at her desk when she developed a severe ache at the back of her head. This was so excruciating that she passed out. Witnesses did not note any shaking of limbs, and she came around within a minute. She vomited twice en route to the hospital and complained of double vision. Her medical history includes polycystic kidney disease (PKD) and hypertension. She is taking ramipril and bendroflumethiazide for hypertension. She does not smoke or drink alcohol. Her sister also has PKD. She did experience a similar but much less severe headache 2 weeks ago but put it down to strain from using a new work computer.

Examination

This woman is oriented, moving her limbs, and speaking appropriately. On neurological examination, there is no limb weakness, and reflexes are present and symmetrical. Plantar responses are flexor. She has a ptosis on the left with the eye depressed and abducted. The pupil is dilated and unreactive to light. There is some mild neck stiffness and photophobia. Her cardiorespiratory and abdominal examinations are unremarkable. Observations: temperature 36.4°C, blood pressure 162/85 mmHg, heart rate 78 beats/min, respiratory rate 18/min, SaO_2 98% on room air.

🔎 INVESTIGATIONS

		Normal range
White cells	4.0	$4–11 \times 10^9$/L
Haemoglobin	12.1	13–18 g/dL
Platelets	220	$150–400 \times 10^9$/L
Sodium	141	135–145 mmol/L
Potassium	5.0	3.5–5.0 mmol/L
Urea	6	3.0–7.0 mmol/L
Creatinine	98	60–110 µmol/L

❓ QUESTIONS

1. What is the diagnosis, and how might you confirm this?
2. What would be the appropriate management?

ANSWERS

This woman presents with a sudden onset of a severe occipital headache with evidence of a third nerve palsy, as shown by the ptosis and eye position. Sudden severe headache is characteristic of subarachnoid haemorrhage (SAH). The third nerve palsy suggests damage to the nerve secondary to rupture of a posterior communicating artery berry aneurysm on the left side. She also has features of mild meningeal irritation and vomiting, which can occur in significant bleeds. There is no suggestion of an infective or vasculitic process, as her history is acute, she is afebrile, and has normal inflammatory markers.

An urgent CT head scan is required to determine the presence of subarachnoid blood, which will show up as hyperdense areas in the basal cisterns, possibly extending to the fissures and sulci. Oedema and mass effects may also be detected. With small bleeds, a CT scan can fail to show blood in the basal cisterns. In this case a lumbar puncture for cerebrospinal fluid (CSF) sampling must be performed. It is recommended that a lumbar puncture be performed after 12 hours from the onset of headache, since, if red blood cells are present in the CSF, they will start to break down and release enough bilirubin and oxyhaemoglobin into the CSF to be detected. It is important to take four samples and to send them to the laboratory immediately, protected from light (which causes oxyhaemoglobin to form more quickly). The laboratory will spin the samples down to ensure no blood cells contaminate the analysis, which might have come from a 'traumatic' tap. Once spun down, the CSF can be visually inspected. In significant bleeds the CSF can appear yellow, which is the xanthochromia from the bilirubin and oxyhaemoglobin; however, this is not a reliable confirmation, and spectrophotometry should be performed, which reliably detects the presence of these pigments. It is no longer appropriate to send three consecutive samples to detect a decrease in the number of red cells.

Further assessment involves identifying the cause of the bleed. In this woman a berry aneurysm is suspected. The most common next investigation would be either a CT angiography or MR angiography. They are non-invasive methods, but the gold-standard method is catheter angiography.

Most subarachnoid haemorrhages (80%) are caused by the rupture of a saccular aneurysm. They occur at the bifurcations of arteries. Their formation is associated with adult polycystic kidney disease, Marfan's syndrome, neurofibromatosis type 1, Ehlers-Danlos syndrome, and pseudoxanthomata elasticum.

In this case the patient has a history of PKD. The most common type is autosomal dominant PKD of which there are two defective genes (*PKD1*, 80% of cases, and *PKD2*, 20%). Hypertension is common, and chronic renal failure develops by the age of 70 years in those with PKD1. If there is a family history of SAH, the likelihood of SAH in autosomal dominant PKD is much higher than if there is no history of SAH.

If a CT head scan confirms a bleed, the main priorities in acute care are to ensure the patient is stable and to arrange urgent referral to a neurosurgical unit. In this case the patient's Glasgow Coma Scale (GCS) score is 15/15, but she has neurological signs, and her GCS must be monitored frequently to detect any deterioration in consciousness level that might necessitate airway protection. A frequent full neurological examination should also be part of management to detect progression of symptoms, which might indicate further bleeding, oedema, or hydrocephalus. She should therefore be managed in an intensive care unit. She should be started on nimodipine, which prevents vasospasm and has been shown to improve outcomes after aneurysmal bleeds.

Strong analgesia should be given for the headache. Hyponatraemia can develop with SAH, and abnormal clotting can exacerbate the bleed; hence both must be monitored and corrected.

Urgent referral for surgical intervention to treat a suspected aneurysm is required. The two main methods are either surgical clipping or endovascular coil embolisation.

? KEY POINTS

1. In suspected SAH, a CT head scan can be normal.
2. A lumbar puncture should be performed at least 12 hours after the onset of headache.
3. Those with SAH and PKD should warrant screening for cerebral aneurysms in other family members with PKD.

CASE 48: BLISTERS AND ITCHY SKIN

History

A 72-year-old man has presented to his general practitioner (GP) after noticing large blisters developing over his arms, legs, and lower abdomen. Some have burst and are uncomfortable. This condition started about 5 days ago. He is otherwise completely well, although he relates that he has had itchy skin for the last couple of months. He is not on any medications.

Examination

There were tense blisters mostly over the arms and legs but also involving the groin and abdomen. Some of the blisters appear clear, but others are bloodstained. A few blisters have burst, leaving an erythematous, moist base. His mouth shows no abnormalities. A cardiorespiratory and abdominal examination is normal. Observations: temperature 37.1°C, blood pressure 146/72 mmHg, heart rate 74 beats/min, respiratory rate 15/min, SpO_2 100% on room air.

? QUESTIONS

1. What is the most likely diagnosis?
2. How would you further investigate and manage this patient?

DOI: 10.1201/9781003241171-48

ANSWERS

The features of tense blisters with a preceding history of pruritus are characteristic of bullous pemphigoid. There are a number of blistering conditions, and the differential diagnoses should include pemphigus vulgaris (generally presents as more superficial erosions and associated more often with oral mucosal lesions) and porphyria cutanea tarda (bullae are on sun-exposed areas).

Bullous pemphigoid is an autoimmune disease caused by auto-antibodies against the hemidesmosomes that link the dermal and epidermal layers. Thus splitting of these layers forms subepidermal blisters, which are tense. It mostly occurs in older people and affects men more frequently than women. There are other forms of bullous pemphigoid, including nodular, vesicular, generalised, urticarial, and erythrodermic.

The diagnosis is made by skin biopsy. Direct immunofluorescence shows immunoglobulin G (IgG) deposition along the basement membrane. An initial assessment must be made of how severe the blistering is and the extent of denuded areas from burst blisters. In those with more severe blistering with exposed areas from burst blisters, there is an increased chance of infection and dehydration, so good skin care and adequate hydration must be maintained. There is an associated mortality risk in those who present with generalised disease and who are older, female, or have co-morbidities. This man is systemically well, but blistering is widespread, so systemic corticosteroids are required. Patients usually respond within 2 weeks. The initial duration of treatment can be up to 9 months, so patients should be provided a steroid treatment card and counselled for potential adverse reactions, especially for signs of adrenal insufficiency. Interval monitoring of blood pressure, HbA1c, body weight, and eye examinations should be arranged. Furthermore, immunisation update, gastric protection with a proton pump inhibitor, and osteoporosis prevention with calcium and vitamin D supplementation and bisphosphonates should be provided. Bullous pemphigoid is usually a self-limiting disease but may last from months to years.

> **? KEY POINTS**
>
> 1. Bullous pemphigoid is an autoimmune disease presenting with tense blisters often preceded by pruritus.
> 2. Bullous pemphigoid is associated with considerable mortality in those who are older and with co-morbid disease.

CASE 49: POSTOPERATIVE HYPOTENSION

History

A 65-year-old man underwent an elective abdominal aortic aneurysm repair. He had a medical history of heart failure secondary to ischaemic heart disease, chronic renal impairment, and type 2 diabetes mellitus.

Postoperative Complications

Postoperatively this man developed acute abdominal pain and became hypotensive with a systolic blood pressure between 55 and 60 mmHg. He was given fluid resuscitation and required noradrenaline to keep his blood pressure elevated. His blood pressure remained low for about 30 minutes before it responded to fluids and vasopressors. He was oliguric. A haemoglobin from the blood gas machine was 5.5 g/L. He was taken to surgery to repair a leak in the aortic graft and transfused 6 units of blood perioperatively. He remained oliguric for 24 hours until his renal function was repeated on day 3.

INVESTIGATIONS

	Pre-op	Day 1 post-op	Day 3 post-op	Normal range
Na	138	131	129	135–145 mmol/L
K	4.8	5.8	6.5	3.5–5.0 mmol/L
Urea	15	28	32	3.0–7.0 mmol/L
Creatinine	140	280	335	60–110 µmol/L

? QUESTIONS

1. What is the cause of this man's acute renal impairment?
2. What is the management of acute renal failure and hyperkalaemia?

DOI: 10.1201/9781003241171-49

ANSWERS

The most likely cause of the renal impairment is renal failure secondary to hypovolaemia from an acute haemorrhage. The patient also has existing renal impairment, diabetes, and coronary artery disease, all of which make him more at risk of renal hypoperfusion.

Acute kidney injury (AKI; previously known as acute renal failure) is defined as an acute decline in glomerular filtration rate (GFR) from the baseline. The exact rise varies between guidelines, but a useful guide to the presence of AKI is a rise of >1.5 times the baseline creatinine. Urine output can be increased, decreased, or absent. The presence of AKI is associated with increased mortality.

The main causes of AKI can be usefully categorised into pre-, intrinsic, and post-renal. The main pre-renal cause is impaired blood flow to the kidneys from hypovolaemia, haemorrhage, dehydration, or sepsis. Intrinsic renal causes include nephrotoxic drugs, interstitial nephritis, or glomerular disease. Outflow obstructions from stones, enlarged prostate, or masses are post-renal causes.

By day 3, this patient has developed hyperkalaemia and worsening renal function. Initial investigation should be directed at determining a diagnosis (in this case, the most likely cause is hypovolaemia from an acute haemorrhage) and treating complications. Renal ultrasound is useful, as it will determine whether there is an obstructive cause.

Immediately after the operation the patient did receive fluid resuscitation and vasopressor support, but his kidneys were not perfused adequately for at least 30 minutes. Urgent management was to stop the haemorrhage and transfuse with blood products. Now the focus should be on maintaining euvolaemia to ensure intravascular volume is adequate to perfuse the kidneys. In this case, optimising cardiac output and volume status presents an additional challenge in view of his pre-existing renal impairment and heart failure. A crystalloid such as 0.9% saline is acceptable. The exact volume of replacement should be decided on parameters such as mean arterial pressure, cardiac index, and other invasive monitoring available. The use of vasopressors and inotropes may be required to maintain renal perfusion pressures. Caution with intravascular volume replacement is necessary, as the patient already has a history of heart failure, and overfilling can impair cardiac function further. Invasive monitoring of central venous pressure, central venous saturations, and cardiac index is therefore required in the setting of an intensive care unit.

An ECG should be performed to identify any rhythm abnormalities associated with hyperkalaemia (Figure 49.1). ECG signs of hyperkalaemia are tenting of the T waves, loss of P waves, widening of the QRS complex, ventricular tachycardia (VT), or ventricular fibrillation (VF). In this case, the ECG showed absent P waves; a wide QRS complex; and tall, tented T waves. Treatment is required if the potassium level is above 6.0 mmol/L with ECG changes. Initial treatments include administration of 10 mL of 10% calcium chloride or gluconate to stabilise the cardiac membrane. The effects are temporary, and treatment can be repeated after 10 minutes. Intravenous insulin and dextrose should be administered to drive potassium intracellularly. This can lower potassium levels by about 0.5–1 mmol/L and last up to 2 hours. Therefore, it may often need to be repeated.

If acidosis, pulmonary oedema, refractory hyperkalaemia, or uraemia is present, renal replacement therapy is indicated. Renal replacement therapy in the acute setting is generally by continuous venovenous haemofiltration (CVVHF). Other modes include continuous venovenous haemodiafiltration (CVVHDF) and continuous venovenous haemodialysis (CVVHD). CVVHF is preferred to dialysis in most acutely ill patients, as they tend to have

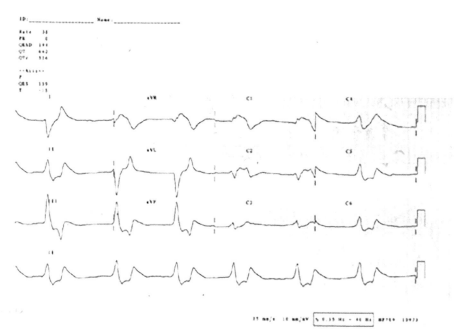

Figure 49.1 An arterial blood gas should be done to determine whether a metabolic acidosis is present. A chest x-ray can help to identify pulmonary oedema.

haemodynamic instability and co-morbidities such as heart failure, which makes tolerating rapid fluid transfers difficult.

Once the underlying cause is removed, the majority of patients with AKI will make a good recovery, although many may never recover full renal function. A small minority will require lifelong renal replacement therapy.

? KEY POINTS

1. Acute renal failure is represented by an acute rise in creatinine and can be caused by several processes. It is essential to diagnose the likely cause and target treatment to this.
2. Renal replacement therapy becomes necessary if there is refractory hyperkalaemia, uraemia, pulmonary oedema, or acidosis.

CASE 50: DROWSINESS BORDERING ON COMA

History

A 78-year-old man was found unrousable in bed by his daughter and has been brought to the emergency department. In the last 2 weeks he was prescribed oral amoxicillin by his general practitioner for a presumptive chest infection. Despite the treatment, he became increasingly lethargic and drowsy, taking to his bed in the past few days. He has had type 2 diabetes for 15 years and is taking metformin and gliclazide. His other medications include lisinopril for hypertension, aspirin for a previous transient ischaemic attack (TIA), and atorvastatin. He does not drink alcohol or smoke.

Examination

This man looks unwell. His mucous membranes appear dry, and he has cool peripheries. His jugular venous pulse (JVP) is not visible, and heart sounds are normal. He has inspiratory crackles and bronchial breathing in the right base. His abdominal examination is normal. His reflexes are normal. Pupils are equal and reactive to light. His score on the Glasgow Coma Scale is 8/15 (does not open eyes, localises to pain, makes incomprehensible sounds). A chest x-ray shows right basal consolidation. An ECG shows sinus tachycardia. Observations: temperature 38°C, blood pressure 98/60 mmHg, heart rate 112 beats/min, respiratory rate 30/min, SpO_2 90% on room air.

🔍 INVESTIGATIONS

		Normal range
White cells	19.0	
Neutrophils	16	
Haemoglobin	17.0	
Platelets	400	
Sodium	156	
Potassium	6.1	
Urea	18	
Creatinine	210	
Chloride	95	
C-reactive protein	288	
Bilirubin	15	
Alanine aminotransferase	34	
Alkaline phosphatase	79	
Albumin	56	
Glucose	37	
Ketones	0.3 mmol/L	
Arterial blood gas on room air:		
pH	7.30	
pO_2	7.5	
pCO_2	3.0	
Lactate	4.0	
HCO_3	16	
Urinalysis	++++ glucose, + protein, no blood, no nitrites or leucocytes, trace ketones	

❓ QUESTIONS

1. What is the diagnosis?
2. How should this patient be managed?

ANSWERS

This man is in a hyperosmolar hyperglycaemic state (HHS) and is showing signs of rapid deterioration towards unconsciousness.

HHS is characterised by severe hyperglycaemia (typically a plasma glucose level >35 mmol/L) and hyperosmolality (serum osmolality >320 mosmol/kg), which can be assessed from 2[Na+] + 2[K+] + [urea] + [glucose]. In this case, the serum osmolality works out to be 379 mosmol/kg. The patient has a mild metabolic acidosis, but significant ketoacidosis is not present (pH >7.3 and ketones <1 mmol/L). This condition mostly occurs in those with type 2 diabetes, in contrast to diabetic ketoacidosis, which occurs in type 1 diabetes. However, the distinction is not absolute, and up to a third of cases can present with both elements.

Precipitants of this condition are usually infection (pneumonia and urinary tract infection are the most common). Other acute stressors such as myocardial infarction, cerebrovascular accident, and surgery can trigger the condition. Significant dehydration, which accompanies this condition, exacerbates electrolyte abnormalities and can cause acute kidney injury. In this case it is likely that the patient has a severe community-acquired pneumonia that has precipitated this state.

The approach to any critically ill person should start with ABCDE (airway, breathing, circulation, disability, exposure). Each step should consist of an assessment and appropriate management before moving on to subsequent stages. This approach is a logical way of thinking through and dealing with an acutely ill person. This approach is part of the IMPACT (Ill Medical Patient's Acute Care and Treatment) method that is recommended by the Joint Royal Colleges of Physicians Training Board. The patient should be managed in a high-dependency area that allows continuous monitoring and early intervention.

This man's airway is at risk owing to his low Glasgow Coma Scale (GCS) score. Early involvement of an anaesthetist or critical care physician is required to provide appropriate airway management. If airway obstruction is detected, basic techniques to keep the airway open (head tilt and chin lift or jaw thrust) with or without airway adjuncts (oropharyngeal or nasopharyngeal airways) should be used until help arrives. The tachypnoea is a response to the metabolic acidosis from acute kidney injury secondary to dehydration and sepsis. Auscultation and chest x-ray showed consolidation at the right base. Saturations and the partial pressure of oxygen are low, with a pO_2 of 7.8 kPa without elevated pCO_2 on room air, which are in keeping with type 1 respiratory failure. In the absence of risk factors for hypercapnic respiratory failure, oxygen should be titrated to maintain a target saturation of 94%–98%.

The patient is hypotensive and tachycardic and requires urgent intravenous access and immediate fluid resuscitation. A urinary catheter should be inserted to quantify urinary output. Shock is defined as inadequate tissue perfusion, and several clinical parameters indicate this (e.g. acute kidney injury, hyperlactataemia, reduced consciousness level). Shock is likely to be caused by hypovolaemia from fluid depletion and sepsis. The 12-lead ECG does not show signs of myocardial ischaemia, and his JVP is not visible without signs of pulmonary oedema, so cardiogenic shock is unlikely.

Initial fluid resuscitation includes a fluid challenge with 500 mL of normal saline given over less than 15 minutes. The patient is likely to be severely dehydrated and sodium depleted and will require large volumes of fluid replacement. However, frequent review of fluid balance, volume, and electrolyte status is required to strike the balance of timely reversal of acute kidney injury, maintenance of electrolyte balance, and to avoid precipitating acute pulmonary oedema. In general, the first 2 L of normal saline can be given over the first 2 hours. Aim for a reduction in osmolality of 3–8 mosmol/kg/hour to avoid precipitating cerebral oedema and pontine myelinolysis. This requires a sodium reduction <10 mmol/L in 24 hours, maintaining potassium within the normal range, and glucose reduction at a rate of 4–6 mmol/L/hr. In the first 24 hours, blood glucose should be maintained at 10–15 mmol/L to avoid hypoglycaemia. Insulin should not be routinely started in HHS unless there is evidence of kentonaemia (>1 mmol/L) or ketonuria (2+ on dipstick), and it should always start after adequate intravenous fluid resuscitation. Potassium level is likely to decrease as the acidosis improves and the intravascular volume increases.

Community-acquired pneumonia is likely the precipitant of this HHS, and intravenous antibiotics should be started without delay. A review of drug history is important in acute kidney injury, and metformin and ramipril should be withheld initially and dosing of medications, if applicable, should be adjusted according to renal function. HHS is a hypercoagulable condition, and thromboprophylaxis is required.

> ### ❓ KEY POINTS
>
> 1. HHS is a serious complication that occurs most commonly in elderly people with type 2 diabetes.
> 2. A common trigger for this is infection.
> 3. Coma is rare but is more likely in those presenting with severe hypernatraemia.

CASE 51: ANXIETY WITH GRAVES' DISEASE

History

A 29-year-old woman has been brought to the emergency department by her husband. He is worried that she is unwell and has been getting worse over the last few days. She describes feeling her heart beating rapidly, difficulty catching her breath, feeling very anxious, hot, sweating a lot, generally weak, and confused. She had varicose vein surgery 5 days ago but had not gone back to work as a schoolteacher because of her symptoms. She was diagnosed with hyperthyroidism secondary to Graves' disease 6 months ago. She was on carbimazole but stopped taking it a week before her surgery, as she was getting a rash. She is taking no other medications. She does not smoke or drink alcohol.

Examination

This young woman is agitated. She feels warm to the touch and has a bounding regular pulse. She appears mildly dehydrated. Her jugular venous pulse (JVP) is low, and there is an ejection systolic murmur over the apex. Respiratory, abdominal, and neurological examinations are unremarkable. She is mildly disorientated in time and place. An ECG shows a sinus tachycardia, and a chest a-ray has no abnormal features. Observations: temperature 39.0°C, blood pressure 178/85 mmHg, heart rate 110 beats/min, respiratory rate 24/min, SaO$_2$ 98% on room air.

INVESTIGATIONS

		Normal range
White cells	5.1	4–11 × 10^9/L
Haemoglobin	11.9	13–18 g/dL
Platelets	340	150–400 × 10^9/L
Sodium	142	135–145 mmol/L
Potassium	4.3	3.5–5.0 mmol/L
Urea	7	3.0–7.0 mmol/L
Creatinine	92	60–110 µmol/L
Thyroid-stimulating hormone	Undetectable	0.4–4.0 mIU/L
Free T4	6.7	0.8–1.5 ng/dL
Free T3	310	0.2–0.5 ng/dL

QUESTIONS

1. What is the most likely diagnosis?
2. What should be this patient's immediate management?

ANSWERS

This woman presents with symptoms and signs characteristic of a thyroid storm. Thyroid storm is an extreme form of thyrotoxicosis. Thyrotoxicosis is defined as the presence of excessive thyroid hormone from any cause (Graves' disease, toxic multinodular goitre, drug side effects, excessive thyroid replacement). The point at which thyrotoxicosis becomes a thyroid storm can be based on criteria such as those devised by Burch and Wartofsky (see Table 51.1). Criteria are based on the presence of thermoregulatory dysfunction, central nervous system effects, gastrointestinal or hepatic dysfunction, and presence of cardiovascular signs. On this scale a score of 45 or greater is highly suggestive of a thyroid storm.

Thyroid storms are a rare presentation; generally milder forms of thyrotoxicosis are more common. Thyroid storms can be triggered in those with a background of hyperthyroidism who have been exposed to stressors such as surgery, severe infection, trauma, myocardial infarction, or pregnancy. It can also occur if an antithyroid drug is discontinued. This patient had a diagnosis of Graves' disease and had been on carbimazole but had stopped it due to side effects. Her recent surgery precipitated thyroid hormone release, which gave rise to her symptoms.

Thyroid storm is life-threatening, as patients can develop seizures, coma, or heart failure. The goal of treatment is to stop thyroid hormone production and limit its peripheral effects. Initial management starts with an assessment of the patient using the ABCDE approach. In this case she does meet Burch and Wartofsky criteria for a thyroid storm; however, in reality, whether she has thyrotoxicosis or storm, the medical management will probably be similar. It should start with supportive therapy, including intravenous fluids, as she is clinically dehydrated. Pyrexia will cause further dehydration, so paracetamol or other cooling measures can be given to manage her temperature. Urgent administration of propyl-thiouracil to stop production of new hormone and stop the conversion of T4 to T3 should be given. The use of steroids such as hydrocortisone is also helpful in reducing the conversion of T4 to T3. In order to reduce the risk of conversion to thyroid hormone, potassium iodide or Lugol's solution is given after approximately 1 hour of the initial thiouracil. This blocks further release of hormone from the thyroid gland. A beta-blocker should also be given to counter the effects on the cardiovascular system (propranolol or metoprolol).

Table 51.1 Scoring System Due to Burch and Wartofsky (1993)

Diagnostic parameters	Scoring points
Thermoregulatory dysfunction	
Temperature (°C)	
37.2–37.7	5
37.8–38.2	10
38.3–38.8	15
38.9–39.2	20
39.3–39.9	25
>= 40.0	30
Central nervous system effects	
Absent	0
Mild (agitation)	10
Moderate (delirium, psychosis, extreme lethargy)	20
Severe (seizures, coma)	30
Gastrointestinal-hepatic dysfunction	
Absent	0
Moderate (diarrhoea, nausea/vomiting, abdominal pain)	10

Diagnostic parameters	Scoring points
Severe (unexplained jaundice)	20
Cardiovascular dysfunction	
Tachycardia (beats/min)	
90–109	5
110–119	10
120–129	15
>= 140	25
Congestive heart failure	
Absent	0
Mild (pedal oedema)	5
Moderate (bibasilar rales)	10
Severe (pulmonary oedema)	15
Atrial fibrillation	
Absent	0
Present	10
Precipitating event	
Absent	0
Present	10

Scoring system: A score of 45 or greater is highly suggestive of thyroid storm; a score of 25–44 is suggestive of impending storm; and a score below 25 is unlikely to represent thyroid storm.
Source: Adapted from Burch, Wartofsky L (1993) Life-threatening thyrotoxicosis: thyroid storm, *Endrocrinol Metab Clin North Am* **22**: 263–77 with permission.

? KEY POINTS

1. Graves' disease is the most common cause of hyperthyroidism.
2. A thyroid storm is an extreme presentation of thyrotoxicosis and is life-threatening if not diagnosed and treated appropriately.

CASE 52: EPISODIC ANXIETY AND HEADACHE

History

A 34-year-old woman attended the emergency department complaining of a severe generalised pounding headache. There is no vomiting, visual disturbance, or other neurological symptoms of note, but the headache is associated with anxiety, palpitations, and diaphoresis. The patient reported similar episodes in the last few months that usually last up to an hour. She feels well between episodes and has no other medical problems. She has tried taking paracetamol and ibuprofen for the headaches, but these did not seem to work. She does not drink alcohol or smoke. There are no significant illnesses in her family history.

Examination

The patient appeared sweaty and pale, but there was no tremor. Her cardiorespiratory, abdominal, and neurological examinations are unremarkable except for tachycardia that are regular. There is no sign of meningism. Her heart rate was 120 beats/min and regular, blood pressure 220/110 mmHg, and respiratory rate 22/min. Fundoscopy did not show papilloedema or other hypertensive changes. An ECG shows sinus tachycardia only. A chest x-ray is normal.

🔍 INVESTIGATIONS

White cells	6.1
Haemoglobin	12.1
Platelets	260
Sodium	148
Potassium	4.8
Urea	5.4
Creatinine	78
Thyroid-stimulating hormone	2.4 nmol/L
C reactive protein	<5
Urine beta-hCG	negative

? QUESTIONS

1. What is the differential diagnosis?
2. What would be appropriate management?

ANSWERS

This patient describes intermittent episodes of palpitations, sweating, and headache associated with hypertension. These features raise the possibility of an underlying phaeochromocytoma. Other diagnoses to consider are hyperthyroidism (may present with tremor and weight loss but her thyroid-stimulating hormone [TSH] is normal), carcinoid syndrome (also episodic, but the predominant symptoms are intense flushing, diarrhoea, and wheeze), anxiety attacks (diagnosis of exclusion), and recreational drugs (amphetamines and cocaine can mimic the features of an episode).

In phaeochromocytoma these symptoms are due to the episodic release of catecholamines from the tumour. Phaeochromocytomas arise predominantly in the chromaffin cells of the adrenal medulla. They produce adrenaline and noradrenaline. Other sites of tumours include chromaffin cells of the autonomic nervous system (paragangliomas). The surge in catecholamines released by these tumours gives rise to the episodic symptoms and signs (headache, sweating, palpitations, and pallor). Tumours are most often benign; malignancy is more likely to occur in paragangliomas. Most cases are sporadic, but up to 40% of cases are hereditary and occur in multiple endocrine neoplasia (MEN) type 2, von Hippel-Lindau disease, and neurofibromatosis type 1.

Diagnosis is made with a 24-hour urine collection or plasma measurements of metanephrines (also called metadrenaline—the breakdown products of catecholamines). Catecholamines tend to release episodically, but metanephrines are released constantly, and therefore metanephrine measurement is preferred. If the urine or blood test is positive, further investigation is required to identify the source. Imaging by CT adrenals will identify most phaeochromocytomas, as 90% arise from the adrenal gland. However, very small (<0.5 cm) and extra-adrenal ones can still be missed. If the suspicion is high despite negative CT adrenals, iodine-131 metaiodobenzylguanidine (MIGB) scintigraphy can be performed. This will detect a phaeochromocytoma anywhere and is over 90% sensitive and specific.

Treatment aims to block the effects of excess catecholamines on the heart and arteries by initiating alpha-blockers at the initial stage. Phenoxybenzamine is traditionally the preferred choice, but doxazosin is an alternative. The reason to withhold beta-blockers prior to sufficient alpha-blockade is to avoid unopposed alpha-receptor stimulation in the arteries, which will lead to a hypertensive crisis from further vasoconstriction. Excess catecholamines leads to intravascular volume constriction, and intravenous fluid replacement may be required. Once adequate alpha-blockade is established, which may take several days, a beta-blocker can be started to reduce the tachycardic effect of catecholamines. If hypertension is not controlled with alpha- and beta-blockade, a calcium channel antagonist can be added. In a hypertensive emergency, the first-line treatment of choice should be intravenous phentolamine (alpha-blocker). Excess catecholamines can inhibit insulin secretion and increase cellular potassium uptake, and therefore glucose and potassium should be monitored. Once blood pressure is controlled and investigations completed, surgery should be considered. Recurrence is more likely in those with a hereditary cause. If the tumour is benign, surgery has a high cure rate. Malignant tumours have a variable course depending on the timing of diagnosis and treatment modalities.

? KEY POINTS

1. Hypertension secondary to phaeochromocytomas should be controlled with the initiation of an alpha-blocker followed by a beta-blocker.
2. Most cases of phaeochromocytomas are sporadic, but up to 40% of cases are hereditary and occur in MEN type 2, von Hippel-Lindau disease, and neurofibromatosis type 1.

CASE 53: COUGH, FEVER, AND SHORTNESS OF BREATH

History

A 52-year-old man is brought into A&E by ambulance with difficulty breathing and a cough. He noticed symptoms starting a week ago, but they have gotten worse. He had attended a friend's dinner party about 2 weeks ago. He doesn't recall anyone being unwell. He otherwise lives with his partner and works from home. He took the usual precautions during the COVID-19 pandemic, but has not had vaccinations for SARS-CoV2. He has a history of ischaemic heart disease with a coronary artery bypass graft (CABG) 5 years ago. He is an ex-smoker and drinks moderate amounts of alcohol. His body mass index (BMI) is 30 kg/m², and he has treated hypertension and told he has diet-controlled diabetes. On arrival to A&E his pulse rate was 94 bpm, BP 105/64 mmHg, oxygen saturations 90% on room air, RR 24 breaths per minute, and he was noted to have a fever of 38.2°C. On examination, he was alert, with Glasgow Coma Scale (GCS) 15/15, but appearing tired. There was reduced air entry bilaterally with some bilateral crepitations. His jugular venous pulse (JVP) was not visible. The rest of the examination was normal.

A chest x-ray (CXR; Figure 53.1) was undertaken:

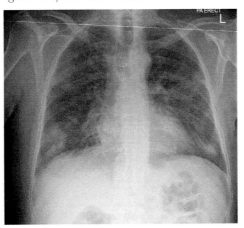

Figure 53.1

A CT chest scan (Figure 53.2) was requested:

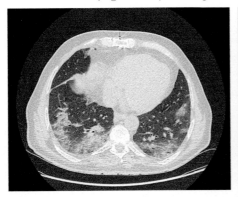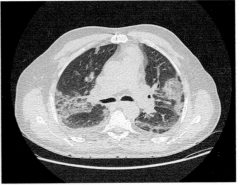

Figure 53.2

DOI: 10.1201/9781003241171-53

ABG showed:

pH 7.36, pO$_2$ 8.4 kPa, pCO$_2$ 3.8 kPa, lactate 3.0 mmol/L, HCO$_3$ 22 mmol/L

Blood tests showed:

- Hb 124 g/L, WCC—low lymphocyte count CRP 105 mg/L Procalcitonin 0.05 ng/mL
- Creatinine 64 umol/L, Urea 4.1 D-dimer Troponin 317
- Bilirubin 7, ALP 76, AST 76 GGT 40

? QUESTIONS

1. What is the likely diagnosis?
2. How would you manage this patient?

ANSWERS

1. The typical symptoms with CXR appearances make COVID-19 disease a likely diagnosis. The CXR shows patchy airspace shadowing in both lung fields, which is in keeping with an atypical pneumonia. An elevated CRP and lymphopenia is characteristic of a viral infection, including COVID-19. It is common to get associated mild transaminitis and low-level raised troponins, which is a marker of disease severity. The procalcitonin is low, indicating a bacterial infection or superinfection is unlikely at this stage. The CT chest confirms the findings of the CXR and helps to rule out other causes for presentation. Other respiratory infections should be considered, including pulmonary emboli and heart failure, but the constellation of symptoms, signs, and investigations makes COVID-19 the most likely diagnosis.

   COVID-19 (coronavirus disease 2019) is caused by the SARS-CoV-2 virus. It first emerged in late 2019 in Wuhan Province, China. It is a zoonotic disease presumed to originate from bats; however, the natural reservoir remains unknown. It has caused a worldwide pandemic. Common presenting symptoms are respiratory but can affect many organ systems, including the heart, gastrointestinal, and renal systems. It has a high mortality rate in elderly people and those with co-morbidities such as obesity, diabetes, hypertension, and immunosuppression. Diagnosis is made from polymerase chain reaction (PCR) of viral RNA isolated from nasopharyngeal swabs. The use of rapid antigen tests are in widespread use, but are not as sensitive as PCR for the detection of the virus. A CT chest can be helpful to diagnose COVID-19 pneumonitis or its associated complications, including pulmonary emboli.

   About a third of people are asymptomatic, but the majority of patients develop a mild course of disease, often beginning with a cough and fever for the first 5–7 days which then might subside and symptoms resolve, but in some the host response to the disease manifests with an abnormal overactive immune response that does not effectively clear the virus. Hypoxia develops, which can lead to multi-organ failure characterised by a cytokine storm. Typically, this occurs from day 8–10 from symptoms.

2. Treatment is focused on organ support and sepsis management. Most patients can be managed on medical wards with supplemental oxygen. Oxygen should be titrated to target saturations (>94% in most patients without risk of hypercapnia). If hypoxaemia is unresponsive to supplemental oxygen, non-invasive ventilation with continuous positive airway pressure (CPAP) can be used, with intubation performed if required. Organ failure and acute respiratory distress syndrome (ARDS) can develop in COVID-19 and should be managed appropriately with supportive care on intensive therapy unit (ITU). Currently licenced specific treatment in selected patients with COVID-19 includes early use of steroids and remdesivir (a viral RNA polymerase inhibitor). Vaccines developed in late 2020 continue to be effective measures in preventing hospitalisations and deaths from severe disease.

? KEY POINTS

1. COVID-19 is caused by a novel coronavirus called SARS-CoV-2, which is distinct from previous severe acute respiratory syndrome (SARS) or Middle East respiratory syndrome (MERS).
2. Severe cases become apparent around day 8–10, when the immune system fails to clear the virus and becomes overactivated.

CASE 54: SHORTNESS OF BREATH FOLLOWING A FALL

History

A 24-year-old woman has been brought to the emergency department by her friends after she developed breathing difficulties while playing football. She noticed some chest pain after a heavy tackle when she landed on her left side. The pain worsened over a few minutes, with associated increasing shortness of breath.

Examination

This young woman looks unwell. She is sweaty, visibly short of breath, and in pain. The right side of her chest wall is not moving and is hyperresonant to percussion. On auscultation there is reduced air entry on the right side. Tracheal deviation to the left is also noted. Her blood pressure is 110/90 mmHg and pulse 115 beats/min. A chest x-ray has been performed (Figure 54.1).

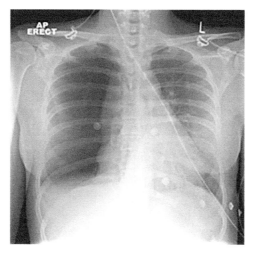

Figure 54.1

? **QUESTIONS**

1. What is the diagnosis?
2. What is shown by the x-ray?
3. How should this condition be managed?

ANSWERS

The symptoms and signs are consistent with a tension pneumothorax: reduced air entry, resonance to percussion, and deviation of the mediastinum to the other side.

Tension develops when air accumulates during inspiration and is not released during expiration. This situation can result from disruption of the pleura and surrounding tissue so that a one-way valve is created, resulting in air only flowing in and not out. With each breath this causes a progressive build-up of air and thus pressure within the pleural cavity, resulting in compression of the lung tissue and surrounding mediastinal structures. It is thought that blood flow to the heart becomes restricted from compression to the superior vena cava, as well as compressing the atria and ultimately the ventricle causing tamponade. Cardiac output falls, and cardiogenic shock ensues. Tracheal deviation is therefore a relatively late sign. Hypotension is an ominous sign.

This is a medical emergency, and immediate decompression is required. Decompression is achieved by inserting a 14-gauge cannula into the pleural space at the second intercostal space and midclavicular line. Enough trapped air can then escape through the cannula to relieve the positive pressure in the chest and allow cardiac filling with improved cardiac output. Meanwhile a chest drain should be inserted.

The diagnosis of a tension pneumothorax is based on a clinical examination, and treatment should be started before a chest x-ray is arranged. A tension pneumothorax can occur with any type of pneumothorax, whether the cause is spontaneous, secondary to underlying pulmonary disease, or caused by traumatic injury from blunt or penetrating injury to the chest wall. In this scenario what makes a tension pneumothorax most likely is the rapidity of the onset of signs with worsening chest pain. The diagnosis can, however, be less clear-cut and present with a more insidious course until the patient is in extremis.

This patient's chest x-ray shows a large, right-sided pneumothorax with some mediastinal deviation. As mentioned earlier, treatment of a tension pneumothorax should be immediate, so a chest x-ray like this should never be obtained! In this case, the patient required a chest drain to be inserted for 48 hours, and the lung gradually re-expanded. She was advised to avoid contact sport for 6 weeks and that she should never dive, as a pneumothorax while diving could be fatal.

? KEY POINTS

1. Tension pneumothorax, although rare, is a medical emergency. Immediate recognition of signs and urgent needle decompression are required. Do not wait for a chest x-ray.
2. Any cause of pneumothorax can result in a tension pneumothorax.

CASE 55: A LADY WITH FATIGUE

History

A 19-year-old student has been brought to the emergency department after her mother found her in bed drowsy and unable to get up unaided. She is fatigued but does not complain of any other problem. However, her mother is extremely concerned about her small amount of food intake. She is a high achiever, and she is obsessed with running. Lately she has been feeling unwell, generally tired and dizzy, but managing to go to university.

Examination

This girl's score on the Glasgow Coma Scale is 14/15 (opening eyes to command, moving limbs spontaneously, coherent speech). She looks very thin, with prominent bony structures and fine body hair. She refused to be weighed due to concerns of being overweight. She has had amenorrhoea for 6 months. She is not taking any medications and does not smoke or drink alcohol. An ECG demonstrates a sinus bradycardia. Observations: tympanic temperature 36°C, heart rate 40 beats/min, blood pressure 90/60 mmHg, SpO_2 98% on room air.

🔍 INVESTIGATIONS

White cells	3.5
Haemoglobin	10.5
Platelets	170
Sodium	130
Potassium	3.0
Urea	5
Creatinine	30
Bilirubin	8
Alanine aminotransferase	48
Alkaline phosphatase	82
Albumin	30
Corrected calcium	2.0
Phosphate	0.6
Magnesium	0.5
Urine beta-hCG	Negative

❓ QUESTIONS

1. What is the diagnosis?
2. What would be your immediate management plan?

DOI: 10.1201/9781003241171-55

ANSWERS

This lady has anorexia nervosa. This is a psychiatric diagnosis characterised by restriction of food intake leading to a significant impact on physical health, intense fear of gaining weight, and altered body image. There are other subtypes, which include 'restricting' calorie intake or 'binge eating/purging' behaviours, which can include laxative, diuretic, or enema use.

Approximately 90% of patients with anorexia nervosa are female, with the onset highest during late adolescence. However, male patients tend not to present for treatment; hence the number of cases in this group is significantly under-detected. There is a tendency for other mood disorders and obsessive-compulsive behaviour traits to manifest. The exact cause of anorexia nervosa is not known, but it is thought to have a genetic basis as well as environmental and other social influences.

A heart rate of 40 beats/min and blood pressure of 90/60 mmHg indicate she is haemodynamically unstable. Her electrolyte abnormalities show hyponatraemia, hypocalcaemia, hypomagnesaemia, and hypophosphataemia. She therefore requires high-dependency care with emphasis placed on haemodynamic stability and intense electrolyte monitoring for refeeding syndrome. Metabolic alkalosis can occur with diuretic abuse and/or induced vomiting.

The patient's underlying mental status may prohibit effective nutritional rehabilitation. Early psychiatry input is essential to support diagnosis, manage psychiatric co-morbidities, and if required, assist in the ethical assessment of treatment refusal. In most cases oral feeding should be attempted initially, and some patients may prefer nasogastric feeding. Total parenteral nutrition should be avoided if possible due to a higher risk in exacerbating refeeding syndrome. This syndrome is more likely to occur in conditions of electrolyte imbalance and is characterised by fluid shifts causing delirium, respiratory, or cardiac failure, as well as gastric dilatation, making feeding even more difficult. Other potential complications are progressive neuromuscular dysfunction and prolonging of the QT interval. Thus, refeeding must be done carefully with close observation and monitoring of electrolytes and clinical condition. A dietitian is essential to determine the number of calories per day, as well as supplementation of vitamins and minerals.

If life-threatening arrhythmias are present from low potassium, more concentrated amounts can be given, but this would be through central venous access. Magnesium and calcium levels often need to be corrected before potassium levels become normal, and continuous ECG monitoring is required. Hyponatraemia should be corrected carefully to avoid precipitating cerebral oedema, seizures, and central pontine myelinolysis.

> **? KEY POINTS**
>
> 1. Anorexia nervosa can present with life-threatening medical emergencies and has a high mortality compared to other psychiatric diagnoses.
> 2. Refeeding syndrome is a potential serious complication of feeding in anorexia nervosa where there are electrolyte imbalances.

CASE 56: HAEMATURIA AND FLANK PAIN

History

A 25-year-old Chinese man attends the emergency department complaining of a constant dull pain in his lower back and passing red blood in his urine since he woke up this morning. He had no dysuria or fever or preceding trauma. He is generally fit and well, working as a teacher. He takes no regular medications and has no significant medical history. He does not smoke or drink alcohol. There is no family history of relevance. His only other complaint was of cold-like (coryzal) symptoms for the past few days.

Examination

There are no significant findings on examination. His blood pressure is 125/65 mmHg. His flank pain settled with analgesia, with improvement in the haematuria spontaneously following 48 hours of observation.

❓ QUESTIONS

1. What is the differential diagnosis?
2. How should this patient be further investigated?
3. How should this patient be followed up?

ANSWERS

The key findings here are frank/macroscopic haematuria and flank pain. Important differential diagnoses to consider are renal stones, urinary tract infection, glomerulonephritis, trauma, renal tract malignancies, benign prostatic hypertrophy, and iatrogenic causes from interventions on the renal tract. The history, examination, and investigations provided exclude most of these causes, except for glomerulonephritis.

The history of a recent upper respiratory tract infection accompanying the previously noted features suggest immunoglobulin A (IgA) nephropathy is the most likely diagnosis. Other differential diagnoses to consider are IgA vasculitis, post-streptococcal glomerulonephritis, and thin glomerular basement membrane disease. Renal manifestations of IgA vasculitis are the same histologically as IgA nephropathy, but IgA vasculitis is characterised by clinical features including purpuric rash, abdominal pain, gastrointestinal bleeding, arthralgia, and peripheral oedema. As part of the full workup, other blood/serological tests should be performed to rule out other causes of glomerular disease, including complement C3 and C4, anti–glomerular basement membrane (GBM), antinuclear cytoplasmic antibodies (ANCAs), antinuclear antibodies (ANAs), chronic hepatitis, and HIV serologies.

IgA nephropathy is the most common glomerular disease worldwide. It occurs most commonly in males (2:1) ages between 20 and 30 years, with a predilection of affecting Asian and European White origins. Most cases are sporadic, but it can be secondary to HIV infection or chronic liver disease. Cases can present in several ways. About half of all cases present as in this case, with frank haematuria and flank pain after an upper respiratory or gastrointestinal infection. A third of patients present with mild proteinuria and microscopic haematuria as an incidental finding as part of other investigations. Up to 10% of patients present with nephrotic syndrome or an acute, rapidly progressive glomerulonephritis (oedema, hypertension, haematuria, and renal failure) or malignant hypertension.

The definitive diagnosis is made with renal biopsy. The timing of renal biopsy varies and is dependent on the case severity at presentation and the subsequent renal function and degree of proteinuria at follow-up. IgA nephropathy is caused by the deposition of IgA in the glomerular mesangium. Sometimes immunoglobulin G (IgG) and complement can also deposit on the mesangium, and this is associated with more severe disease. As this patient is normotensive, has preserved renal function, and has only mild proteinuria, there is no immediate requirement to start drug treatment.

Treatment can be divided into renal supportive and immunosuppressive therapies. The main renal supportive drugs are angiotensin-converting enzyme inhibitors (ACEIs) or angiotensin II receptor blockers (ARBs), and they are initiated when a patient develops hypertension or proteinuria (>0.5 g/day). Immunosuppression is considered in those with persistent proteinuria >1 g/day despite maximum tolerated doses of ACEIs or ARBs and controlled blood pressure. A 6-month course of corticosteroids is considered first-line immunosuppressive treatment. The role of fish oil (omega-3-acid ethyl esters) may have a role in selected patients. The patient in this case should undergo renal specialist follow-up. Urinalysis, renal function, and blood pressure should be checked at least six-monthly.

? KEY POINTS

1. IgA nephropathy is the most common glomerular disease worldwide.
2. IgA nephropathy can have a varied presentation ranging from an incidental finding to nephrotic syndrome or acute progressive glomerulonephritis.
3. Definitive diagnosis is by renal biopsy, but most cases do not require this unless there is significant proteinuria, persistent haematuria, or renal impairment.

CASE 57: BRADYCARDIA AND MALAISE

History

A 74-year-old man has been referred to the emergency department following an assessment by his general practitioner (GP), who found him to be unable to get out of his chair and with a slow heart rate of 30 beats/min. He has had a bout of diarrhoea and vomiting over the past couple of days.

Examination

On arrival an ECG is performed (Figure 57.1). A chest x-ray shows cardiomegaly but clear lung fields. His jugular venous pulse (JVP) is visible 3 cm above the sternal angle with occasional cannon waves. He has dry mucous membranes. He has a midline sternotomy scar. The apex beat is displaced and the impulse diffuse. Heart sounds show a soft pansystolic murmur at the apex. On chest auscultation there are no crackles. Abdominal examination is normal. His ankles are not swollen. He cannot lift his legs off the bed and is generally weak. He has ischaemic heart disease, having had a coronary artery bypass graft 1 year ago. His other medical history is hypertension, hypercholesterolaemia, type 2 diabetes, gout, benign prostatic hyperplasia (BPH), and congestive heart failure. He has had no chest pains over the last year, although his exercise tolerance is limited to 40 metres on the flat, and he has difficulty going up a flight of stairs due to breathlessness. He lives on his own in a flat, mobilising with a frame. He is on aspirin, bisoprolol, ramipril, spironolactone, bumetanide, atorvastatin, omeprazole, metformin, and allopurinol. He has no allergies. He does not smoke or drink alcohol. Observations: temperature 36.4°C, blood pressure 156/78 mmHg, respiratory rate 18/min, SaO$_2$ 94% on room air.

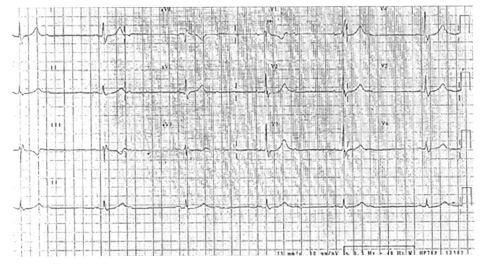

Figure 57.1

DOI: 10.1201/9781003241171-57

INVESTIGATION

		Normal range
White cells	10.0	$4–11 \times 10^9$/L
Haemoglobin	13.3	13–18 g/dL
Platelets	199	$150–400 \times 10^9$/L
Sodium	145	135–145 mmol/L
Potassium	7.9	3.5–5.0 mmol/L
Urea	32	3.0–7.0 mmol/L
Creatinine	245	60–110 µmol/L
Venous blood gas pH	7.35	7.35–7.45

? QUESTIONS

1. What is the main life-threatening abnormality, given the biochemistry and ECG findings?
2. What are the potential causes of this?
3. How should this patient be further investigated and treated?

ANSWERS

The main blood abnormality is hyperkalaemia. The level of 7.9 mmol/L is very high, and this is the likely cause of his muscle weakness and complete heart block (shown on the ECG and indicated clinically by the bradycardia and cannon waves). He also has renal impairment.

Hyperkalaemia has several causes, so focusing investigations is crucial to allow timely and appropriate treatment. Often a combination of underlying problems may be the cause. In this case the most important to consider are:

- Worsening chronic kidney disease
- Drug-related
- Obstruction
- Cardio-renal syndrome
- Volume depletion

Urgent investigations should include a renal ultrasound scan to look for obstruction causing hydronephrosis. It will also help to assess renal size and give an indication as to whether there is likely to be pre-existing chronic renal impairment. A venous blood gas will show if there is metabolic acidosis. Although the patient has congestive heart failure, he has no signs of it at present. He is likely dehydrated from the recent diarrhoea and vomiting.

The patient is on multiple medications that can cause hyperkalaemia either directly or indirectly. Spironolactone is a potassium-sparing diuretic and can raise potassium in some people who are sensitive to this drug. Ramipril can cause hyperkalaemia, and in states of volume depletion from recent diarrhoea and vomiting, this is exacerbated. Bumetanide, a loop diuretic, will exacerbate volume depletion but tend to lower serum potassium. Heart failure is linked to renal impairment: the relationship is complex, and it is known that one exacerbates the other. This phenomenon is termed cardio-renal syndrome.

Management should be based on the immediate need to lower his potassium level and treat his complete heart block. An assessment should be made of haemodynamic stability. If the patient shows signs of hypotension or heart failure or reduced consciousness, he should be given atropine 500 μg intravenously to try to increase the heart rate. Further doses can be administered to a maximum of 3 mg. Isoprenaline infusion is a useful drug to use. If these measures do not work, he will need initiation of transcutaneous pacing with a view to inserting a temporary pacing wire.

Ten per cent calcium chloride or gluconate should be given intravenously as soon as possible. Calcium works by stabilising the cardiac sarcolemmal membrane, but its effects wear off in minutes, so repeated doses may be necessary. Intravenous insulin/dextrose should be commenced to drive the potassium into cells; repeated doses are often required. The patient is clinically dehydrated, and fluid resuscitation should also be administered; normal saline is an appropriate fluid. A fluid challenge can be administered to determine the effect on blood pressure and urine output. He has a history of congestive cardiac failure, so careful fluid resuscitation is important. To help assess fluid balance, a central venous line may be required. The patient should be admitted to the intensive care unit or coronary care unit for continuous cardiac monitoring. If potassium is not improving with insulin/dextrose and fluid resuscitation, he requires renal replacement therapy.

Once potassium levels start to come down, his rhythm may return to normal. Also his renal function should improve with fluids, as this episode is likely to have been precipitated by dehydration from a recent illness made worse by medications. Metformin, aspirin, and allopurinol should all be discontinued in the short term. Metformin is associated with lactic acidosis in the setting of significant renal failure.

Significant hyperkalaemia is defined as K >6 mmol/L, while moderate hyperkalaemia is 5–6 mmol/L; all levels above 6 should be treated. Treatment should be given between 5 and 6 if associated with ECG changes. ECG changes in hyperkalaemia include early changes (peaked T waves, shortening of the QT interval and ST segment depression). Later changes are widening of the QRS complex, prolongation of the PR interval, and eventual loss of P waves. Eventually the QRS complex widens further to appear as a sine wave. At this point ventricular fibrillation or asystole can follow. However, any arrhythmia can be caused, including various degrees of atrioventricular (AV) block. A comprehensive "Clinical Practice Guidelines Treatment of Acute Hyperkalaemia in Adults" is published by The Renal Association and regularly updated, providing useful advice on the diagnosis and management of hyperkalaemia in both the community and hospital settings in the UK.

> **? KEY POINTS**
>
> 1. Hyperkalaemia is life-threatening. When found, an ECG must be performed in all cases.
> 2. Hyperkalaemia has many causes, and the diagnosis is based on a focused history, examination, and appropriate investigations.

CASE 58: SWELLING OF LOWER LIMBS

History

A 63-year-old man was referred to the ambulatory clinic for further assessment because of progressive bilateral lower limb swelling in the last month. He has also noticed that his urine is more frothy than usual. He does not complain of cough, shortness of breath, or chest pain. There is no weight loss or fever. He has no significant medical history. He drinks wine on occasion, does not smoke, and is not on any medications. He is a retired painter and decorator.

Examination

This man has pitting oedema up to the thighs. His SpO_2 is 95% on room air, blood pressure is 135/80 mmHg, pulse 72 beats/min and regular, and respiratory rate 12/min. A cardiovascular, respiratory, abdominal, and neurological examination are within normal limits.

INVESTIGATIONS

White cells	8.0	$4-11 \times 10^9$/L
Haemoglobin	15.0	13–18 g/dL
Platelets	350	$150-400 \times 10^9$/L
Sodium	128	135–145 mmol/L
Potassium	3.7	3.5–5.0 mmol/L
Urea	5.8	3.0–7.0 mmol/L
Creatinine	130	60–110 µmol/L
Bilirubin	8	5–25 µmol/L
Alanine aminotransferase	30	8–55 IU/L
Alkaline phosphatase	52	42–98 IU/L
Albumin	21	35–50 g/L
Urinalysis	Protein ++++, no blood	
24-hour urinary protein	11 g	

12-lead ECG: Normal sinus rhythm

Chest x-ray: Normal

Echocardiogram: Normal LV systolic and diastolic function. No valvular abnormalities detected. Normal right ventricular size and function.

? QUESTIONS

1. What is the most likely diagnosis?
2. How should the patient be further investigated and managed?

ANSWERS

The presence of oedema, hypoalbuminaemia (<30 g/L), and significant proteinuria (>3.5 g in 24 hours) are diagnostic of nephrotic syndrome. This condition is associated with hyperlipidaemia and a hypercoagulable state. Urine protein:creatinine test is a useful alternative to 24-hour collections. A ratio of >300 mg/micromole is diagnostic for nephrotic-range proteinuria.

In nephrotic syndrome the disruption of the glomerular filtration barrier, which is made up of fenestrated endothelium of the capillary, basement membrane and the podocytes foot processes, leads to protein leak from the glomeruli. The protein loss and compensatory production by the liver lead to several complications. Peripheral oedema is a direct result of hypoalbuminaemia from the loss of albumin and sodium retention in the collecting ducts. The increased thrombotic risk is due to a loss in anticoagulation factors (anti-thrombin III, protein C and S) and increased synthesis of procoagulant factors and platelet activation. The liver also increases the production of very low and low-density lipoproteins, resulting in hypercholesterolaemia and hypertriglyceridaemia and accelerated atherosclerosis. Increased infection risk is due to the loss of immunoglobulins and complements. This is further exacerbated by the immunosuppressive drugs sometimes used to treat nephrotic syndrome.

Nephrotic syndrome is a presentation feature for several renal disease, and patients are at risk of end-stage renal disease and associated complications. Therefore, careful clinical assessments and investigations are required to establish the underlying cause and to target the management accordingly. This man does not have another cause for oedema (e.g. cardiac failure) or hypoalbuminaemia (e.g. protein-losing enteropathy or chronic liver disease). The patient's age, ethnicity, and co-morbidities at presentation are helpful in narrowing down the extended list of possible causes, which include:

- Primary glomerular disease: minimal change disease, focal segmental glomerulosclerosis, membranous nephropathy
- Systemic disease: diabetic nephropathy, multiple myeloma, immunoglobulin A (IgA) nephropathy, systemic lupus erythematosus (SLE), amyloidosis
- Infections: hepatitis B virus (HBV), hepatitis C virus (HCV), HIV, post-streptococcal, syphilis, endocarditis
- Malignancy: Hodgkin's lymphoma and other solid organ tumours
- Drugs: gold, penicillamine, non-steroidal anti-inflammatory drugs (NSAIDs), captopril, lithium
- Other rare causes: Alport's syndrome, Fabry's disease, nail-patella syndrome

The most common causes in adults are membranous nephropathy, focal segmental glomerulosclerosis, and diabetic nephropathy. The cause of nephrotic syndrome in adults often requires a renal biopsy for a definitive diagnosis. Therefore anyone presenting with features of nephrotic syndrome should be referred to a renal specialist.

General care of a patient with nephrotic syndrome includes (i) careful diuresis to manage peripheral oedema and to avoid exacerbating acute kidney injury; (ii) attention to cardiovascular risk prevention, including optimal lipid and blood pressure control; (iii) advice on immunisations to prevent infections; (iv) prophylactic anticoagulation during inpatient stay; and (iv) attention to nutrition due to negative protein balance and salt retention state.

In this case, the patient was found to have membranous nephropathy. A renal biopsy was required to make the diagnosis. Following supportive treatment with fluid restriction and renal function monitoring, as well as improving the patient's blood glucose and cholesterol levels, he made a good recovery.

? KEY POINTS

1. Nephrotic syndrome is associated with infections, venous and arterial thromboses, and dyslipidaemia.
2. Nephrotic syndrome in adults often requires a renal biopsy to determine the underlying cause.

CASE 59: HAEMOPTYSIS AND SHORTNESS OF BREATH

History

A 67-year-old man has presented to the emergency department with a week history of increasing shortness of breath and cough with small amount of blood with his sputum. He has also noticed that his urine has become cola coloured. He came back from Spain 4 weeks ago and has felt very fatigued since. He smokes 15 cigarettes per day and drinks 4 pints of beer per week. He is on no medications. He works as a gardener.

Examination

This man has bibasal inspiratory crackles in the mid/lower zone on auscultation of the chest. The rest of the cardiorespiratory, abdominal, and neurological examinations are normal. Observations: temperature 37.3°C, blood pressure 165/85 mmHg, heart rate 85 beats/min, respiratory rate 24/min, SpO_2 92% on room air.

🔍 INVESTIGATIONS

		Normal range
White cells	9.2	
Haemoglobin	11.0	
Platelets	400	
Sodium	138	
Potassium	5.0	
Urea	19	
Creatinine	280	
CRP	72	
INR	1.1	
Urine dipstick	Blood +++ Protein ++	
Urine microscopy	Red cell casts	

A chest x-ray shows bilateral diffuse airspace opacification mostly in the lower zones.

Echocardiogram: normal left and right ventricular function. No valvular abnormality detected.

? QUESTIONS

1. What is the likely diagnosis?
2. How would you manage this patient?

ANSWERS

This man presents with clinical and radiological features of diffuse alveolar haemorrhage and acute kidney injury secondary to glomerulonephritis, which is indicated by the presence of red cell casts. This is consistent with pulmonary-renal syndrome, an autoimmune-driven process that occurs in association with rapidly progressive glomerulonephritis and diffuse alveolar haemorrhage.

Immediate management should focus on ensuring he is receiving adequate oxygenation. He should be closely monitored in a high-dependency area for the requirement for further respiratory support such as mechanical ventilation and correction of any coagulopathy. Fibreoptic bronchoscopy and bronchoalveolar lavage are helpful in confirming the presence of pulmonary haemorrhage. A renal opinion should be sought as a matter of urgency to establish the underlying diagnosis with a renal biopsy.

The main causes of pulmonary-renal syndrome are anti-neutrophil cytoplasmic antibody (ANCA)–associated vasculitis and anti–glomerular basement membrane disease (anti-GBM or Goodpasture's disease). ANCA-associated vasculitis includes granulomatosis with polyangiitis (previously Wegener's granulomatosis), microscopic polyangiitis, and eosinophilic granulomatosis with polyangiitis (previously Churg-Strauss syndrome). In ANCA-associated vasculitis, clinical features include skin manifestations (purpuric rash or pyoderma gangrenosum), arthritis, scleritis, malaise, fever, peripheral neuropathy, and mononeuritis multiplex. Upper airway complications such as epistaxis, destruction of nasal cartilage, and hoarse voice occur mostly in granulomatosis with polyangiitis, but they can also affect other forms of ANCA-associated vasculitis. By contrast, arthritis, myalgia, and neuropathy are usually absent in Goodpasture's disease, and haemoptysis is the predominant presenting symptom. Less common causes of pulmonary-renal syndromes are lupus nephritis, cryoglobulinaemic vasculitis, and post-streptococcal glomerulonephritis. In all cases, investigations should therefore include anti-GBM antibody, ANCA, antinuclear antibody (ANA), C3 and C4, cryoglobulins, chronic viral hepatitis serology, and anti-streptolysin O titre. In 30%–50% of cases those with Goodpasture's disease will also test positive for ANCA. ANA and serum complement C3 and C4 are useful to investigating lupus nephritis, infection, endocarditis, or cryoglobulinaemia. Chronic hepatitis B and C are associated with cryoglobulinaemic vasculitis.

First-line therapies involve pulsed methylprednisolone (1 g intravenously for 3 days) followed by prednisolone (1 mg/kg/day orally, maximum dose 80 mg/day), tapered gradually over 3 months, and cyclophosphamide. In the most severe cases plasma exchange is also required. Rituximab has been shown to be effective in selected cases. Cigarette smoking is strongly discouraged in all patients. If renal impairment is severe enough to require haemodialysis at presentation, there is usually a low likelihood of renal recovery.

? KEY POINTS

1. Recognition of a pulmonary-renal syndrome with early diagnosis and treatment offers the best chance of renal function recovery.
2. Pulmonary haemorrhage is potentially fatal and requires urgent treatment with oxygen, corticosteroids, plasma exchange, and cyclophosphamide.

History

A 29-year-old man attends the ambulatory clinic with a 7-day history of headache. It started during a busy weekend fitting ceiling lights in his new home. This headache is described as left-sided, constant in the fronto-temporal region, with 5/10 in severity. It is not associated with nausea and vomiting, photophobia, lacrimation, dizziness, seizure, weakness, or loss in sensation. He has no history of chronic headache or weight loss. His family is concerned about the associated left eyelid droop and the persistent headache despite simple analgesia. He is not a smoker. He drinks 21 units of alcohol per week and does not report any recreational drug use. There is no family history of note.

Examination

This man looks well. Cardiorespiratory, abdominal, and peripheral nervous system examinations are unremarkable. There is no lymphadenopathy. There is a partial ptosis of the left eyelid associated with a miosis of the left pupil that is not responsive to light. The ptosis is mild and appears to disappear when asked to look up. Swinging light test is negative. There is no cranial nerve abnormality detected. Plantar response is flexor bilaterally. Observations: temperature 36.9°C, heart rate 87 beats/min, respiratory rate 12/min, SpO_2 99% on room air.

🔍 INVESTIGATIONS

White cells	4.0
Haemoglobin	14.2
Platelets	287
Sodium	139
Potassium	3.9
Urea	4.2
Creatinine	65
CRP	<5
INR	1.0

A chest x-ray shows a normal cardiothoracic ratio and normal lung fields.

? QUESTIONS

1. What is the likely diagnosis, and how would you confirm this?
2. How would you manage this patient?

ANSWERS

This man presents with a history of moderate headache with an ipsilateral Horner's syndrome, which is characterised by miosis and partial ptosis. The other features of Horner's syndrome are anhidrosis and enophthalmos. This contrasts with third nerve palsy, where the ptosis is complete and the pupils are dilated. Anhidrosis only occurs when the defect is preganglionic (central) because innervation to the sweat gland by the sympathetic chain is proximal to the superior cervical ganglion. The term 'preganglionic' encompasses the sympathetic pathway from the brainstem to the C8/T1 spinal cord and then the T1 nerve root to the superior cervical ganglion. As it runs through several structures, the possible lesions are brainstem stroke, spinal cord tumours/demyelination/syrinx, Pancoast's tumour, cervical rib, mediastinal mass, cervical lymphadenopathy, thyroid mass, and complications from neck surgery. Postganglionic lesions distal to the superior cervical ganglion include carotid artery dissection/aneurysm or mass within the middle cranial fossa. Enophthalmos, or posterior displacement of the eye due to paralysis of the upper and lower eyelid tarsus muscle, is rare and difficult to recognise. In this case, the site of the lesion is likely postganglionic. The onset of the symptoms was associated with activities that hyperextend the neck, which is a risk factor for carotid artery dissection. This was later confirmed on CT angiogram (for head and neck), which demonstrated a small dissection 2 cm distal to the origin of the left internal carotid arteries.

Carotid artery dissection is a common cause of stroke in people older than 40 years. The presentation can vary markedly, ranging from subtle symptoms and signs (like this case) to retinal infarction, amaurosis fugax, and middle cerebral artery infarction. As a result, presentation and diagnosis are sometimes delayed. Any headache/neck pain that presents with Horner's syndrome requires exclusion of carotid artery dissection. Activities that hyperextend or rotate the neck may cause minor trauma to the artery leading to dissection, which include car accident, contact sports, medical procedures, and daily activities such as ceiling painting. Some connective tissue disorders such as Marfan's syndrome, fibromuscular dysplasia, and Ehlers-Danlos syndrome are predisposed to cervical artery dissection (carotid or vertebral artery dissection). Hyperextension or rotation of the neck can also cause vertebral artery dissection. This presents with occipital headache and/or posterior neck pain +/− posterior circulation ischaemia, which includes brainstem, cerebellar signs, and Horner's syndrome.

Treatment of carotid artery dissection depends on the presence of a stroke, the speed of haematoma expansion in the false lumen, and the site of the dissection. In all cases, a stroke/neurology opinion should be sought. In this case, the patient appears to be stable with no sign of clinical deterioration. The aim is to prevent cerebral ischaemia, and antiplatelets and/or anticoagulants will be required for this indication. Endovascular stents may occasionally be required.

? KEY POINTS

1. The presentation of carotid artery dissection can vary from minor symptoms to a severe stroke, so a high index of suspicion is required, especially in those presenting with headache or neck pain and Horner's syndrome.
2. Horner's syndrome is caused by lesions that disrupt the sympathetic chain. A systematic clinical assessment is required to determine the underlying cause.

CASE 61: KNEE SWELLING AND PAIN

History

A 75-year-old man attends the emergency department with severe pain in his left knee. This started 2 days ago, and he is now unable to walk. He has a history of heart failure for which he has been taking lisinopril, bisoprolol, aspirin, atorvastatin, and indapamide. Recently furosemide was added to his treatment because of increasing ankle oedema.

Examination

This elderly man's left knee is swollen with evidence of an effusion, and it is erythematous and tender to the touch and very painful on any movement. No other joints are affected. There is no skin rash. A sample of fluid aspirated from the knee is initially bloodstained; then straw-coloured turbid fluid is obtained. Observations: temperature 37.3°C, blood pressure 142/86 mmHg, heart rate 90 beats/min, respiratory rate 20/min. A knee x-ray reveals no bony abnormalities.

INVESTIGATIONS

Synovial fluid:
- White cells   10567/mm³ (75% neutrophils)
- No organisms seen
- Negatively birefringent crystals seen

QUESTIONS

1. What is the most important differential diagnosis?
2. What is the most likely diagnosis?
3. How would you manage this patient?

DOI: 10.1201/9781003241171-61

ANSWERS

This man presents with a very painful acute monoarthritis associated with erythema, which is most likely a result of acute gout or septic arthritis. The latter needs to be excluded urgently. Raised white cells in synovial fluid can occur in both gout and septic arthritis. The presence of negative birefringent crystals is diagnostic of gout. The lack of organisms seen in microscopy is reassuring, but the synovial fluid needs to be sent for culture, as gout and septic arthritis can rarely coexist. The other differential diagnosis is acute calcium pyrophosphate crystal arthritis (pseudogout), but positive birefringent crystals is seen in the synovial fluid in these cases.

Gout is a condition in which urate crystals deposit within joints causing an inflammatory arthritis. It occurs more commonly in men and increases in incidence with age. Ninety per cent of cases involve one joint, and oligo- or polyarticular involvement tends to present in chronic gout. Uric acid crystals can also deposit in the glomerulus causing tubular and inter-stitial disease as well as uric acid stones. Gout is associated with hyperuricaemia, although elevated levels of serum uric acid do not always result in gout, and it can be elevated for up to 20 years before the onset of gout. Chronic kidney disease and drugs such as diuretics, tacroli-mus, and ciclosporin increase the risk of gout by reducing excretion of uric acid, leading to an elevated serum uric acid level. Some people have tophi from urate deposits on the hands, the helix of the ears, or over extensor surfaces. They are sometimes detectable after 10 years after the first gout attack.

The affected joint should be rested appropriately with application of ice packs. Non-steroidal anti-inflammatory drugs (NSAIDs) are the first-line treatment. If there are contraindications to NSAIDs (e.g. gastrointestinal [GI] bleed from a peptic ulcer), colchicine is an alternative, but it has a slower onset of action. Side effects are common and include diarrhoea, nausea, and vomiting. Dose reduction for colchicine is required in older patients and those with esti-mated glomerular filtration rate <30 mL/min. Statins should be temporary withheld, as drug interactions with colchicine may occur leading to rhabdomyolysis. Treatment with NSAIDs or colchicine should continue for at least 1 week even if symptoms settle early to avoid a rebound attack. If the patient is intolerant to NSAIDs or colchicine, corticosteroids should be used under specialist advice. Intra-articular injection of corticosteroid can be used once septic arthritis is ruled out. Other routes such as oral or intramuscular injections can also be considered. The anti-interleukin-1 drug canakinumab has marketing authorisation as a third-line treatment for gout, but it is not endorsed by the National Institute for Health and Care Excellence (NICE) and is therefore not widely available.

The xanthine oxidase inhibitor allopurinol is indicated for patients experiencing more than one gout attack per year. Other indications include those with tophi, chronic kid-ney disease, transplant-associated gout, renal stones, and in patients who require ongoing diuretics for heart failure. As this man is dependent on diuretics for heart failure, this should be started 7–14 days after the acute gout attack. This is to prevent a gout attack due to a sudden drop in serum uric acid, although this risk appears to be less than previ-ously thought. Allopurinol should not be stopped during an acute attack if the patient is established on this. Allopurinol should be up-titrated monthly, aiming for serum uric acid <300 μmol/L. Febuxostat is an alternative to allopurinol, but it is contraindicated in those with pre-existing cardiovascular disease. Lifestyle factors should be addressed to advice limiting alcohol intake, high-purine foods (seafood and red meat), and drinks with fructose or corn syrup.

🔑 KEY POINTS

1. Gout is a condition in which urate crystals deposit within joints causing an inflammatory arthritis.
2. Gout can have a similar presentation to pseudogout. They can be differentiated by looking at the synovial fluid under a microscope. In gout there are negatively birefringent crystals, whereas in pseudogout there are positively birefringent rhomboid-shaped crystals.
3. Urate crystals may be deposited in the glomeruli and lead to tubular and interstitial disease as well as uric acid stones. High urate levels can also cause a nephropathy and eventually renal failure.

CASE 62: LOWER ABDOMINAL PAIN

History

A 58-year-old man was admitted to the A&E by his general practitioner (GP) for suspected appendicitis. He had complained of lower abdominal pain for several days and had an intermittent fever. The GP felt he was tender in the left lower quadrant and observed his temperature to be 37.8°C. His HR was also 101 bpm. On arrival to A&E his HR was 110 bpm, with a BP of 98/60 mmHg. Respiratory rate was 18 breaths per minute. Oxygen saturation on room air was 96%. On examination he was very tender over the left lower quadrant, but no mass was present. There was no evidence of guarding or rebound tenderness. The patient reported a history of constipation, but no recent change in bowel habit or blood noted in the stools. Apart from a sinus tachycardia, his cardiorespiratory exam was normal. He had a history of diverticulosis with previous lower abdominal pain that subsided spontaneously and hypertension but did not smoke or drink alcohol. The patient only took ramipril for blood pressure control. He had no significant family history. He was a builder by trade.

His blood tests were as follows:

Blood test	Result	Normal range
White cells	13.5	4–11 × 109/L
Haemoglobin	16	13–18 g/dL
Platelets	445	150–400 × 109/L
Sodium	142	135–145 mmol/L
Potassium	4.8	3.5–5.0 mmol/L
Urea	8.0	3.0–7.0 mmol/L
Creatinine	115	60–110 umol/L
INR	1.1	0.9–1.1

? QUESTIONS

1. What is the immediate management of this patient?
2. What investigations would be appropriate to determine the cause?

DOI: 10.1201/9781003241171-62

ANSWERS

1. The patient has signs of sepsis with hypotension and tachycardia. Intravenous access should be obtained and a bolus of crystalloid fluids administered. In addition, bloods should be taken for culture and lactate levels. Broad-spectrum intravenous antibiotics covering gut organisms should be administered as soon as possible after cultures are taken. Oxygen saturations should be targeted to >94% and urine output measured. Early critical care involvement should be instituted if septic shock does not respond to fluid resuscitation. A surgical opinion should also be sought if perforation or an abscess is suspected. A differential diagnosis should include appendicitis, inflammatory bowel disease, or complications from malignancy and in women gynaecological causes. Most cases can be managed conservatively if there are no complications with antibiotics, fluids, and analgesia. Diverticulum can occasionally cause a lower gastrointestinal (GI) bleed if a diverticulum erodes into a vessel.

2. After immediate stabilisation and treatment, an appropriate investigation would be a CT of the abdomen with contrast, as this will aid diagnosis and look for complications such as perforation or abscess formation. The patient's history of diverticulosis makes this the most likely cause in this case. Fifteen per cent of acute presentations will develop complications. Up to 50% of patients develop recurrent diverticulitis. Longer-term complications of repeated bouts of inflammation can include bowel strictures and fistulas.

Diverticulosis is thought to be more common in those with a low dietary fibre diet, obesity, smokers, and increasing age.

KEY POINTS

1. Diverticulitis is mostly managed conservatively with antibiotics and analgesia; however, a minority of cases can present with complications including lower GI bleed, fistulas, perforations, or abscess formation.
2. Diverticulosis is common in Western populations and increases with age.

CASE 63: ABDOMINAL PAIN, BRUISING, AND CONFUSION

History

A 51-year-old woman has presented to the emergency department feeling generally unwell with abdominal pain, bruising, and confusion. Her friend states that she has been complaining of general tiredness, nausea, and joint pains for 2 months. She has a history of hypothyroidism and Sjögren's syndrome. She does not smoke or drink alcohol. There has been no exposure to viral hepatitis or recent travel abroad. Her only prescribed drugs are levothyroxine and Hypromellose eye drops. She has not taken any over-the-counter medications.

Examination

This woman appears unwell with deep yellow sclerae, scratch marks, bruising over her arms and legs, and spider naevi over her chest and back. There is a coarse tremor of her outstretched hands. In her abdomen there is hepatomegaly and evidence of ascites. She is drowsy but easily rousable and obeys simple commands only. Observations: temperature 36.9°C, heart rate 97 beats/min, respiratory rate 18/min, BP 90/65 mmHg, SpO$_2$ 95% on room air.

INVESTIGATIONS

White cells	10.0
Haemoglobin	10.1
Platelets	120
Sodium	132
Potassium	4.5
Urea	12
Creatinine	123
Bilirubin	267
Alanine aminotransferase	3169
Aspartate aminotransferase	3277
Alkaline phosphatase	378
Albumin	28
Prothrombin time	32 seconds

QUESTIONS

1. What is the diagnosis, and how would you manage this patient?
2. What tests would you do to identify the underlying cause?

ANSWERS

This woman presents with evidence of hepatic encephalopathy and coagulopathy consistent with acute liver failure. She requires immediate transfer to the intensive care unit for the optimal management of haemodynamics, coagulopathy, nutrition, metabolic complications such as hypoglycaemia, fluid and electrolyte balance, and hepatic encephalopathy. She is also at risk of infection, gastrointestinal bleeding, acute kidney injury, and cerebral oedema.

Identifying the cause of hepatic failure is important, as it can determine further therapy and also the likelihood of suitability for liver transplantation. There are several causes of acute liver failure, which include viral (hepatitis A, B, and D), idiosyncratic drug-related liver injury (e.g. anti-tuberculous antibiotics, sulpha-containing drugs, nitrofurantoin, phenytoin, carbamazepine, valproate, flutamide, and amoxicillin-clavulanate), poisoning (e.g. paracetamol, methotrexate) metabolic (Wilson's disease), and portal vein thrombosis.

Initial assessments of acute liver failure therefore include alcohol history, risk factor for viral hepatitis, drug history including herbal and recreational drug use, and history of deliberate self-harm and poisoning. Abdominal ultrasound scan with Doppler is required to assess the liver for size, lesion, evidence of portal hypertension, and to look for portal vein thrombosis. Several laboratory tests are specifically required to assess the severity and to investigate the underlying cause of the acute liver failure. This includes prothrombin time/international normalised ratio (INR); glucose; ammonia; lactate; electrolytes; creatinine; liver enzymes; full blood count; serum immunoglobulin concentrations; and viral hepatitis screen, including hepatitis A, B, C, and E, Epstein-Barr, herpes simplex and varicella zoster viruses, and HIV. Autoimmune panel, including antinuclear antibody (ANA), antimitochondrial antibody (AMA), anti–smooth muscle antibody (SMA), and antibodies to liver-kidney microsomal (anti-LKM) and liver cytosol (LC). If appropriate, paracetamol level and pregnancy test in women of childbearing age should also be obtained. In this case, it would be reasonable to request a CT brain to exclude intracranial pathologies that may coexist.

Cerebral oedema arising from hepatic encephalopathy is the leading cause of death in acute liver failure. Patients with grade 3 or above (somnolence, confusion, or coma) hepatic encephalopathy should be sedated and intubated to protect the airway and to control for arterial $paCO_2$ to 4.5–5 KPa using mechanical ventilation. Patients should be nursed head up at 30 degrees. Haemodialysis should be considered if ammonia >150 μmol/L (if not for other indications) and to maintain sodium between 145 and 155 mmol/L. Ongoing surveillance for sepsis and frequent monitoring of fluid balance, electrolytes, creatinine, coagulation profile, and glucose are required to treat any emergent complications. The gut is the main site of ammonia production, which drives hepatic encephalopathy. Therefore, constipation should be prevented with lactulose, rifaximin, or enemas. Discussion with a tertiary referral centre experienced in the management of acute liver failure should be made. The decision for liver transplantation can be very difficult and is based on the probability of spontaneous hepatic recovery. Various criteria exist to guide decisions on transplantation. For instance, the King's College Hospital criteria for non-paracetamol aetiologies include a prothrombin time of >100 seconds (independent of grade of encephalopathy) or any three of the following: age <10 or >40; aetiology (non-A, non-B hepatitis, drug reactions); duration of jaundice before onset of encephalopathy >7 days; prothrombin time >50 seconds; bilirubin >300 μmol/L.

In this case, the history of autoimmune disease and preceding features suggest autoimmune hepatitis (AIH) could be the underlying cause. AIH can present insidiously with months of mild abdominal discomfort, pruritus, arthralgia, and general malaise. A simplified diagnostic score for AIH is used to aid diagnosis, taking into account histological findings and serology, including elevated immunoglobulin G and presence of ANA, SMA, anti-LKM, and LC. The presence of AMA suggests an alternative diagnosis of primary biliary cholangitis instead of AIH. Autoantibodies can be negative in 20% of AIH cases.

Treatment for AIH involves corticosteroids and immunosuppressants. Treatment is recommended for those with serum aspartate aminotransferase levels greater than 10-fold the upper limit of normal, or twice the upper limit of normal with histology indicating non-inflammatory changes. The first-line combination therapies for AIH are prednisolone and azathioprine. Liver transplantation in AIH is associated with a 5-year patient survival of between 80% and 90%. In some cases, AIH can recur in transplanted livers.

 KEY POINTS

1. Acute liver failure requires intensive care and referral to a liver transplant centre.
2. AIH can present in a variety of ways: asymptomatic with raised aminotransferases but no fibrosis, or inflammation found on biopsy, to the rare presentation of acute hepatic failure.

CASE 64: JAUNDICE AND PRURITIS

History

A 62-year-old woman is referred to ambulatory care for assessment after presenting to her general practitioner (GP) complaining of malaise and change in skin colour in the last 2 weeks. In the last 12 months, she has been increasingly fatigued and has a generalised itch that is worse in the palms and feet, especially in the evenings. She has not had any abdominal pain, vomiting, melaena, change in bowel habit, or weight loss. She has hypothyroidism and takes levothyroxine but no other medications including herbal or recreational drugs. There was no travel history. She reports a positive family history of coeliac disease which affects her mother and her two sisters. She does not smoke and she usually drinks 1–2 units of alcohol per week.

Examination

This woman is icteric. Xanthelasmas are noted around both eyes. There are spider naevi around her upper torso and arms and palmar erythema on her hands. Her cardiovascular and respiratory examinations are normal. The abdomen is distended with a palpable but non-tender liver at 4 cm below the right costal margin. A bilateral pitting oedema up to mid-shins is noted. There is no tremor or lymphadenopathy. She is fully orientated and responds appropriately. Observations: temperature 36.2°C, heart rate 68 beats/min, blood pressure 134/72 mmHg, SpO$_2$ 97% on room air.

INVESTIGATIONS

White cells	9.1
Haemoglobin	10.7
Platelets	100
Sodium	132
Potassium	4.0
Urea	5.1
Creatinine	84
Bilirubin	154
Alanine aminotransferase	75
Alkaline phosphatase	834
Gamma-glutamyl transpeptidase	876
Albumin	28
INR	1.5
C-reactive protein	
Total cholesterol	6.8
HDL cholesterol	1.8

? QUESTIONS

1. How would you manage this woman?
2. What is the differential diagnosis?
3. What additional tests would you require to confirm the diagnosis?

DOI: 10.1201/9781003241171-64

ANSWER

This woman presents with cholestatic jaundice as indicated by the raised bilirubin and a marked increase in alkaline phosphatase (ALP) and gamma-glutamyl transpeptidase (GGT). It is important to exclude any associated bacterial cholangitis and primary or metastatic cancer, e.g. pancreatic cancer, cholangiocarcinoma, or liver metastasis. There is no history of biliary colic, drug-induced liver injury, or evidence of bacterial cholangitis (abdominal pain or fever) in this case. An ultrasound abdomen should be requested urgently to exclude any biliary obstruction and focal liver lesions. It can also examine for features of portal vein hypertension, including spleen size and the extent of ascites and also for thrombosis. This woman has clinical features of end-stage chronic liver disease, as evident by the clinical signs and an impairment of liver synthetic function (hypoalbuminaemia and raised international normalised ratio [INR]). She should be admitted to investigate for the underlying cause and to evaluate and to treat any complication resulting from portal hypertension, e.g. a screening oesophagogastroduodenoscopy (OGD) for oesophageal and gastric varices, diuresis, and lactulose/rifaximin to prevent constipation that can precipitate hepatic encephalopathy.

If there is no evidence of mechanical biliary obstruction, further laboratory investigations should include serum immunoglobulins, antinuclear antibody (ANA), antimitochondrial antibodies (AMA), and anti–smooth muscle antibodies (SMAs) to screen for autoimmune causes of cholestatic jaundice, which are primary biliary cholangitis (PBC, previously primary biliary cirrhosis) and primary sclerosing cholangitis (PSC). Viral hepatitis B and C and HIV serologies should be screened for despite the cholestatic picture, as they may coexist and may alter clinical management.

Patients' demographics and co-morbidities are helpful in differentiating PBC and PSC. PBC affects predominantly women in their late 40s to 60s with a female:male ratio of 9:1. It is an autoimmune condition and is associated with personal and family history of autoimmune syndromes such as Sjögren's syndrome, autoimmune thyroid disease, and coeliac disease. The main symptoms for PBC are pruritis, mainly in the palmar-plantar distribution, especially in evenings, and fatigue symptom complex, which consists of mild memory disturbance (independent of encephalopathy), severe fatigue, and autonomic dysfunction (flushing, sweating, and orthostatic symptoms). Laboratory investigations reveal an elevated serum immunoglobulin M. Ninety per cent of PBC patients have positive AMA and 50% have positive ANA, specifically the subset anti-glycoprotein210, anti-Sp100, or anti-centromere antibodies. By contrast, PSC typically affects younger men with a male:female ratio of 2:1. Seventy per cent of cases are associated with inflammatory bowel disease (particularly ulcerative colitis). AMA antibodies are usually absent. ANA and SMA are usually negative or weakly positive only. Magnetic resonance cholangiopancreatography is helpful in differentiating PBC from PSC, as the latter shows multiple segmental strictures and biliary tree dilatation, which is absent in PBC. Liver biopsy is not always required for PBC and PSC when clinical, laboratory, and radiological features are typical. In this case, the more likely diagnosis is PBC. The clinical presentation of PBC can range from incidental finding of raised ALP to end-stage liver failure. Xanthelasma and raised cholesterol are associated with PBC, but the cholesterol components that are raised are typically high-density lipoprotein (HDL) and lipoprotein X, and therefore it is not always correlated with accelerated atherosclerosis. If low-density lipoprotein (LDL) is raised, statin can be used safely, but this requires careful clinical monitoring. First-line treatment for all patients with PBC is ursodeoxycholic acid therapy, which is a choleretic and a cytoprotectant. Cholestyramine is given as an anti-pruritic but is often poorly tolerated, and off-label rifampicin, acting as a pregnane X receptor agonist, is a highly potent alternative. She should be referred to a tertiary liver transplant centre, as the only definitive treatment option for patients with end-stage liver disease is liver transplantation.

🔑 KEY POINTS

1. Cholesterol is often raised in PBC. Statin therapy is not contraindicated.
2. PBC presents with a cholestatic picture, whereas autoimmune hepatitis mainly affects transaminases—although there can be a degree of cross-over between the two conditions. A liver biopsy can be helpful in distinguishing them.

CASE 65: BLEEDING GUMS AND NOSE

History

A 58-year-old man has presented to the emergency department with intermittent nosebleed and bleeding gums for the last 6 hours. He also has a fever, cough with purulent sputum, and shortness of breath, which appeared over the last 24 hours. His past medical history includes psoriasis and hypertension, and his conditions are well controlled on methotrexate, indapamide, and folic acid. He does not smoke or drink alcohol. He has been well prior to the current illness, and his blood test results had been normal a month earlier.

Examination

This man is alert and orientated but lethargic. There is evidence of recent bleeding from the gums, and both nostrils are packed to manage the epistaxis. There is bruising over his arms and legs. No lymphadenopathy is found. Cardiovascular, neurological, and abdominal examinations are unremarkable. On respiratory examination there is reduced air entry at the left base with inspiratory crackles. An ECG shows a sinus tachycardia. Observations: temperature 38.0°C, blood pressure 110/78 mmHg, heart rate 110 beats/min, respiratory rate 24/min, SpO_2 94% on room air.

🔍 INVESTIGATIONS

White cells	1.9
Neutrophils	0.9
Haemoglobin	7.5
Platelets	33
Sodium	135
Potassium	3.5
Urea	11.0
Creatinine	180
INR	1.2
C-reactive protein	99

Chest x-ray: left lower lobe consolidation
ECG: sinus tachycardia

❓ QUESTIONS

1. What are the main abnormalities on the laboratory investigations? How does this account for the clinical picture?
2. What are the possible causes for the abnormalities on the full blood count in this case? How should this be investigated?
3. What should be the management of this patient?

ANSWERS

The full blood count results showed pancytopenia as evidenced by anaemia, leucopenia, and thrombocytopenia. There is acute kidney injury and raised C-reactive protein, most likely consistent with the left lower lobe pneumonia. Of particular concerns are the ongoing bleeding due to thrombocytopenia, neutropenic sepsis, and acute kidney injury.

Pancytopenia is a result of the reduction in haematopoiesis in the bone marrow or increased consumption/destruction of cells. In some diseases such as myelofibrosis, the pancytopenia is due to a combination of reduced production and increased consumption/destruction. Moreover, in patients with multiple co-morbidities, it is possible to have several causes that contribute to pancytopenia. The main causes of reduced haematopoiesis are adverse drug reactions (e.g. chemotherapy), radiotherapy, infections, nutritional deficiency, fibrosis or infiltration of the bone marrow by haematological and non-haematological malignancies, immune destruction leading to aplastic anaemia, and paroxysmal nocturnal haemoglobinuria. The main causes for increased consumption/destruction are hypersplenism and severe sepsis.

The most likely cause for this patient's presentation is methotrexate. It works by inhibiting dihydrofolate reductase, leading to suppression of nucleic acid synthesis in rapidly dividing cells. Concomitant folic acid usually reduces the possibility of bone marrow toxicity, but in this case the renal impairment may have predisposed the myelosuppression by markedly reducing the elimination of methotrexate. Both methotrexate and indapamide should be withheld immediately.

The initial management of this patient involves aggressively treating his bleeding and sepsis. He should be managed in a high-dependency area with reverse barrier nursing. Assessment of his airway, breathing, and circulation is crucial to determine his subsequent management. He will need replacement of red blood cell and platelet transfusion, as he has active bleeding. Clotting profile should also be re-checked and clotting factors replaced if required. Broad-spectrum antibiotics should be started as soon as feasible, preferably before blood culture (or sputum culture) as per local protocol, but this should not be delayed. Continuous haemodynamic monitoring with fluid status assessment will be required to optimise fluid resuscitation. Haematology input would be helpful to guide blood product replacement and further investigations.

As mentioned before, there could be more than one cause of pancytopenia, so further assessments should be conducted. In this case the patient was relatively well and did not report any weight loss or B symptoms prior to the current presentation. There were no lymphadenopathy, splenomegaly, or masses on examination. There was no history of cancer, chronic liver disease, or other connective tissue disease such as systemic lupus erythematosus and rheumatoid arthritis. In all cases, investigations should include viral serology (HIV, hepatitis B/C, Epstein-Barr virus [EBV], and cytomegalovirus [CMV]), haematinics (vitamin B_{12} and folate), reticulocyte count, lactate dehydrogenase, haptoglobin, and blood film. The latter is particularly helpful in narrowing down the differential diagnosis (e.g. leucoerythroblastic appearance suggests bone marrow infiltration or myelofibrosis, and blast cells suggest leukaemia).

Pancytopenia due to vitamin deficiencies usually takes 1 week to recover, but those that are drug induced may take many weeks to recover. Bone marrow biopsy may not be helpful in drug-induced pancytopenia, as it is often non-diagnostic when performed too early. Folinic acid may be helpful in accelerating the bone marrow recovery in methotrexate-induced myelosuppression. Granulocyte colony-stimulating factor can be considered under specialist guidance once haematological malignancy is excluded.

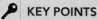 **KEY POINTS**

1. Methotrexate can cause myelosuppression even at low doses, especially in renal impairment. Folic acid is co-prescribed to prevent bone marrow toxicity.
2. Pancytopenia can present as sepsis, bleeding, or both.

CASE 66: PALPITATIONS AND SHORTNESS OF BREATH

History

A 75-year-old woman presented to her general practitioner (GP) with palpitations and exertional shortness of breath. She had been experiencing palpitations intermittently over the last 2 years but had noticed her heart racing more often. She now gets short of breath when going up stairs. She is taking medications for hypertension. She does not smoke or drink alcohol. She is systemically well and has no other significant medical or family history. As her symptoms were getting worse, her GP decided to refer her to the medical admissions unit.

Examination

Her pulse is irregularly irregular with a rate of about 120/min. On cardiovascular and respiratory examination, there is a raised jugular venous pressure (JVP), displaced apex beat, and fine inspiratory crackles at the lung bases, with mild swelling of her ankles. Her blood pressure is 160/75 mmHg. An ECG is shown in Figure 66.1 and a chest x-ray in Figure 66.2. Respiratory rate is normal, and her pulse oximetry is also normal. Her heart rate slowed down slightly following initial treatment in the emergency department, but the examination findings remained unchanged.

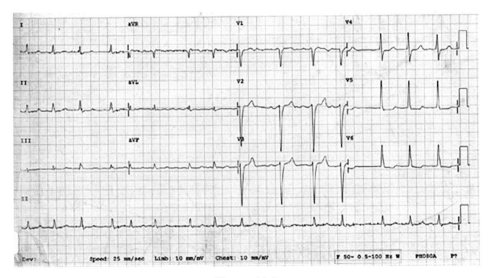

Figure 66.1

DOI: 10.1201/9781003241171-66

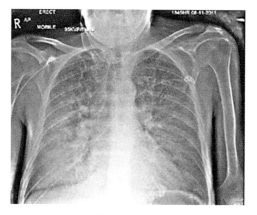

Figure 66.2

? QUESTIONS

1. What is the diagnosis?
2. What are the likely causes?
3. How should this patient be managed?

ANSWERS

This woman has atrial fibrillation (AF) with a fast ventricular response. The ECG shows atrial fibrillation: note that there are no P waves before the QRS complex, which is narrow, and that the heart rate is irregularly irregular. The fast rate and the loss of atrial transport from the fibrillation will impair cardiac function. The basal inspiratory crackles suggest that she has left ventricular (LV) dysfunction. The chest x-ray shows fluffy, interstitial shadowing and prominent upper-lobe blood diversion, suggestive of pulmonary oedema.

Initial management should focus on determining the presence or absence of chest pain, pulmonary oedema, and haemodynamic instability. Hypotension or worsening pulmonary oedema is a sign that she is not tolerating the irregular fast ventricular rates, and she will then need to be cardioverted either electrically or chemically. However, in this case, although the patient does have signs of fluid overload, she is haemodynamically stable and comfortable at rest.

AF becomes more common with increasing age such that more than 10% of those aged over 80 years have AF. The most common causes are hypertension, heart failure, ischaemic heart disease, and valvular disease. Hyperthyroidism is another cause and may not have obvious clinical signs in the elderly.

Initial management should focus on managing immediate complications, controlling the ventricular rate, and considering antithrombotic therapy. She has evidence of congestive heart failure but has a good blood pressure with normal oxygen saturations, and the up-to-date ECG suggests reasonable rate control. Immediate treatment with intravenous diuretics such as furosemide would be recommended to treat pulmonary congestion. According to current evidence and guidance, rate control without rhythm control is a reasonable initial approach. First-line therapy involves beta-blockers or non-dihydropyridine calcium channel blockers. However, this patient has signs of heart failure on clinical examination and on chest x-ray. Commencing with digoxin may be better in this situation, as it is not a negative inotrope. In this case, the patient was loaded with digoxin in the emergency department and then continued on a maintenance dose. She should undergo an echocardiogram to assess LV size and function and any valvular pathology that might underlie her AF.

Concomitantly she should be assessed for stroke risk. Direct oral anticoagulants (DOACs) have now become the preferred anticoagulant to initiate patients on if one or more stroke risk factors are present. Stroke risk can be estimated from a score (CHA_2DS_2VASc: Congestive heart failure, Hypertension, Age ≥75 (doubled), Diabetes, Stroke (doubled), Vascular disease, Age 65–74, and Sex category (female)—see Table 66.1A). A score of 2 predicts a 2.2% per year adjusted stroke risk (see Table 66.1B). This is generally accepted to be the cut-off to starting treatment with an oral anticoagulant provided there are no contraindications.

The main concern with anticoagulants is the risk of bleeding, and an assessment of this risk should be made prior to starting treatment. A bleeding risk score such as HAS-BLED can be used to assess risk (see Table 66.2). Although DOACs are now the anticoagulants of choice, warfarin is still used in specific patient groups (valvular AF, e.g. rheumatic mitral stenosis and enlarged left atrium, presence of metallic valves).

NSAIDs, non-steroidal anti-inflammatory drugs.

Reproduced from 'Guidelines for the management of atrial fibrillation ESC', *Eur Heart J*, 2010, **31**: 2369–429 with permission.

Apart from the initial management of rate control and anticoagulation, longer-term strategies to manage rhythm in AF can be considered if felt it will help related symptoms (e.g. breathlessness,

Table 66.1A CHA$_2$DS$_2$VASc Scoring

Risk factor	Score[a]
Congestive heart failure/LV dysfunction	1
Hypertension	1
Age ≥75 years	2
Diabetes mellitus	1
Stroke/transient ischaemic attack/thromboembolism	2
Vascular disease[b]	1
Age 65–74 years	1
Sex category (female sex)	1

Source: Adapted from 'Guidelines for the management of atrial fibrillation ESC', *Eur Heart J*, 2010, **31**: 2369–429 with permission.

[a] Maximum score is 9 (age may contribute 0, 1, or 2 points).
[b] Vascular disease represents prior myocardial infarction, peripheral arterial disease, or aortic plaque.

Table 66.1B Adjusted Stroke Risk According to the CHA$_2$DS$_2$VASc Score

Score	Adjusted stroke risk (per year)
0	0%
1	1.3%
2	2.2%
3	3.2%
4	4.0%
5	6.7%
6	9.8%
7	9.6%
8	6.7%
9	5.2%

Source: Adapted from 'Guidelines for the management of atrial fibrillation ESC', *Eur Heart J*, 2010, **31**: 2369–429 with permission.

Table 66.2 HAS-BLED Bleeding Risk Score

Letter	Clinical characteristic	Points awarded
H	Hypertension	1
A	Abnormal renal or liver function (1 point each)	1 or 2
S	Stroke	1
B	Bleeding	1
L	Labile INRs	1
E	Elderly (age >65 years)	1
D	Drugs (NSAIDs and antiplatelets) or alcohol (1 point each)	1 or 2

fatigue, reduced exercise tolerance, or palpitations). A trial of sinus rhythm induced by electrical cardioversion can be tried to see if symptoms improve. AF ablation tends to have greater success rates with left atria that are not too enlarged.

🔑 KEY POINTS

1. AF, particularly with a fast ventricular response rate, will lead to a reduced ejection fraction and impaired cardiac function.
2. Rate control is important to ensure that the ventricles fill sufficiently, and medications such as beta-blockers and digoxin may be necessary to achieve this.
3. AF causes stasis of blood within the heart chambers, increasing the risk of embolic stroke. Anticoagulation is often commenced to prevent this, but the risk of bleeding with warfarin and heparin needs to be considered.

CASE 67: SHORTNESS OF BREATH AND PEDAL OEDEMA

History

A 52-year-old man presented to the emergency department because of progressive dyspnoea over 4 weeks. Prior to this he was completely well. He had no history of heart disease, lung problems, or diabetes. He has been told he has high blood pressure but is not receiving any treatment for it. He smokes 10 cigarettes per day and drinks about 4 pints of lager per week.

Examination

The man was noted to be overweight. His jugular venous pulse was elevated. Heart sounds were normal, chest was clear but there was pedal oedema. Observations: temperature 36.5°C, blood pressure 164/84 mmHg, heart rate 150 beats/min, respiratory rate 22/min, SaO$_2$ 96% on room air.

A chest x-ray showed small bilateral pleural effusions and cardiomegaly. An ECG was performed (Figure. 67.1).

Initial Treatment

In the emergency department he was given amiodarone, and during the infusion his heart rate was noted to slow to 70 beats per minute in sinus rhythm. A couple of days later an echocardiogram was performed, which showed moderately impaired left ventricular (LV) function. The patient was commenced on a diuretic and an angiotensin-converting enzyme (ACE) inhibitor was started. When he was euvolaemic, bisoprolol was also commenced.

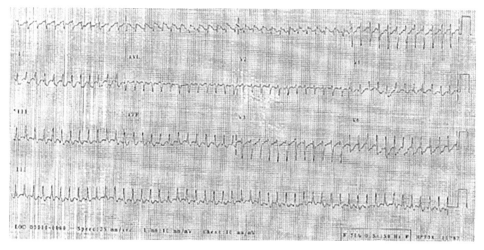

Figure 67.1

? **QUESTIONS**

1. What is the likely diagnosis?
2. How would you manage this patient?

ANSWERS

The ECG shows a regular rate at almost 300/min, but it is difficult to make out the P waves. Differential diagnoses of a supraventricular tachycardia (SVT) include sinus tachycardia, atrial fibrillation and flutter, atrioventricular (AV) nodal re-entry tachycardia (AVNRT), AV re-entry tachycardia (AVRT), and multi-focal atrial tachycardia.

In this case amiodarone was administered to attempt chemical cardioversion, which appeared to be successful in this case.

Management of any SVT depends on the condition of the patient. If the patient shows signs of shock, heart failure, or myocardial ischaemia, then he or she should be electrically cardioverted with a synchronised DC shock.

If the patient is stable, in regular SVT, if there is no contraindication, adenosine can be given, which may terminate the tachycardia if it is an AVRT or AVNRT. If flutter is the underlying rhythm, then rate control is the aim (e.g. beta-blocker or digoxin). In this case although the man was haemodynamically stable, he had mild features of fluid retention, and chemical cardioversion was tried. Fast irregular rates are likely to be atrial fibrillation, and then rate control is the initial treatment of choice with anticoagulation if indicated.

Fast atrial fibrillation or flutter of several weeks' duration can lead to a rate-related cardiomyopathy, which tends to improve with rate control.

KEY POINTS

- Atrial flutter and fibrillation increase the risk of stroke. Anticoagulation should be considered.
- SVT has various causes.
- Immediate treatment is dependent on patient stability. Unstable patients require immediate electrical cardioversion.

CASE 68: SHARP CENTRAL CHEST PAIN

History

A 42-year-old woman has presented to the emergency department with chest pain. It is central, sharp in nature, and made worse by inspiration and by lying down. The pain eases when she sits forward. She had no medical history and is taking no medications. She is a non-smoker and does not drink alcohol. She works as a health care assistant.

Examination

On examination of the precordium there is a rub heard at the left lower sternal edge in systole and diastole. The rest of the cardiorespiratory and abdominal examination is unremarkable. Observations: temperature 37.6 °C, heart rate 98 beats/min, blood pressure 121/72 mmHg, respiratory rate 18/min, SaO$_2$ 100% on room air.

A chest x-ray shows a normal-sized heart and clear lung fields. An ECG shows widespread ST elevation (Figure 68.1).

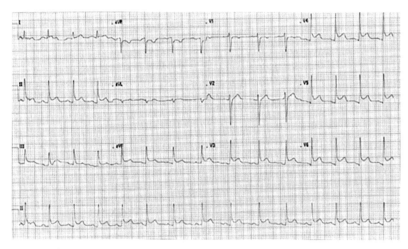

Figure 68.1 Supplied by Dr Stam Kapetanakis.

? QUESTIONS

1. What is the most likely diagnosis?
2. How would you manage this patient?

ANSWERS

This patient's signs and symptoms with the ECG changes are consistent with an acute pericarditis. Viral pericarditis is the most common cause and is associated with coxsackievirus B and influenza epidemics. Other causes include autoimmune diseases and uraemia associated with renal failure.

She should have an echocardiogram, which is usually normal but sometimes shows evidence of a pericardial effusion, which may need to be monitored. A large pericardial effusion can cause cardiac tamponade, and a pericardiocentesis is sometimes required to drain off the fluid.

It is likely that this woman has a viral pericarditis, which is usually a limiting disease process. She will need to rest until the pain settles and should make a full recovery over the following days to weeks. A patient with a high fever (>38°C) or significant underlying medical problems may need to be admitted for monitoring, as he or she may be at risk of developing serious complications. Other blood tests that would be supportive of an acute pericarditis are an elevated CRP and white cell count.

This woman should take a 7-day course of a regular non-steroidal anti-inflammatory drug (NSAID) such as ibuprofen. This will act to reduce inflammation and settle her chest pain. Low-dose colchicine can be used as an adjunct with NSAIDs. Patients who do not respond to an NSAID may need a course of corticosteroid.

Pericarditis can develop in the weeks following a myocardial infarction (Dressler's syndrome). As with other cases of pericarditis, this is usually self-limiting, and administration of an NSAID provides sufficient treatment. The presentation can be mistaken for a pulmonary embolism (sharp chest pain following a recent hospital admission) and so should always be considered following a recent myocardial infarction. In some cases myopericarditis can develop, and this is identified by a mild to moderately elevated troponin level. A subsequent echocardiogram or cardiac MRI can identify any associated myocardial dysfunction.

 KEY POINTS

1. Pericarditis can present acutely or chronically. Pain is usually pleuritic and positional with characteristic ECG changes showing widespread saddle-shaped ST elevation.
2. Most cases of acute pericarditis are viral and self-limiting.

CASE 69: CHEST PAIN WITH FEVER, MALAISE, AND MYALGIA

History

A 45-year-old man has been referred to the medical admissions unit with a 2-week history of fever, malaise, and myalgia, having developed central chest discomfort 4 days ago. He describes the pain as tight, and he was becoming more short of breath on exertion. He has a history of hypertension. He is not on any medications and has no significant family history. He smokes 20 cigarettes per day and drinks 12 units of alcohol per week.

Examination

This man's jugular venous pressure (JVP) is not raised. Heart sounds are normal. The chest is clear to auscultation, with no evidence of peripheral oedema. Abdominal examination is normal. There is no lymphadenopathy, clubbing, or skin rashes. Musculoskeletal examination is normal. An ECG (Figure 69.1) shows less than 1 mm ST elevation in the inferior leads; PR interval normal; QRS complex was of normal duration and morphology. Axis was normal. A chest x-ray shows mild cardiomegaly on a posteroanterior (PA) projection. Lung fields are clear. Observations: temperature 37.8°C, heart rate 101 beats/min, blood pressure 145/62 mmHg, respiratory rate 20/min, SaO_2 98% on room air, blood sugar 5.2 mmol/L.

🔍 INVESTIGATIONS

		Normal range
White cells	13.2	$4-11 \times 10^9$/L
Neutrophils	8.0	$2-7 \times 10^9$/L
Lymphocytes	2.7	$1-4.8 \times 10^9$/L
Haemoglobin	14.4	13–18 g/dL
Platelets	350	$150-400 \times 10^9$/L
Sodium	137	135–145 mmol/L
Potassium	4.2	3.5–5.0 mmol/L
Urea	4.0	3.0–7.0 mmol/L
Creatinine	68	60–110 µmol/L
C-reactive protein	154	<5 mg/L
Troponin-T	1.4	<0.03 µg/L
Arterial blood gas sample:		
pH	7.43	7.35–7.45
pO_2	7.4	9.3–13.3 kPa
pCO_2	3.1	4.7–6.0 kPa
Lactate	2.7	<2 mmol/L
HCO_3	24	22–26 mmol/L
Base excess	+1	−3 to +3 mmol/L
Saturation	87%	>94%

DOI: 10.1201/9781003241171-69

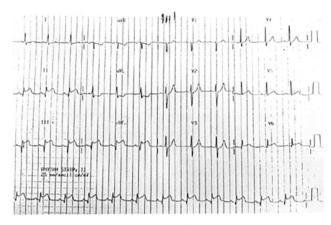

Figure 69.1

? QUESTIONS

1. What are the differential diagnoses?
2. How would you further investigate this patient?

ANSWERS

This man's ECG (Figure 69.1) shows inferior changes with a raised troponin in keeping with myocardial damage. However, the aetiology is not immediately obvious. He presents with a fever and raised inflammatory markers with a prodromal illness. Apart from hypertension, he has no risk factors for ischaemic heart disease. These symptoms fit best with myocarditis. Myocarditis is uncommon, but tends to affect young adults. Acute myocarditis can present mildly, as in this case, or in extremis with cardiogenic shock or sudden death. The causes of myocarditis include infections (viral being the most common—parvovirus B19, adenovirus, coxsackie B, human herpesvirus-6, cytomegalovirus, Epstein-Barr virus, herpes simplex, HIV), autoimmune diseases (e.g. systemic lupus erythematosus, rheumatoid arthritis), and drug-induced (anthracyclines).

The patient is haemodynamically stable, and there is no evidence of heart failure. An echocardiogram will determine whether there is any left ventricular functional impairment. He may well have inferior wall motion abnormalities, as the ECG suggested some inferior changes. It is not uncommon to find regional ST elevation on an ECG in patients with myocarditis. An echocardiogram will also identify any associated pericardial effusion. A sensitive and specific test to help confirm the diagnosis of myocarditis is an MRI with gadolinium enhancement. Typically parts of the myocardium with acute inflammation show elevated T2 signals consistent with myocardial wall oedema. Late gadolinium enhancement can identify areas of inflammation and scar formation consistent with a non-ischaemic pattern (e.g. mid-wall pattern sparing the endocardium). However, in cases of severe myocarditis, a large portion of the myocardium can be affected. In selected cases, endomyocardial biopsy may be required to make the diagnosis and assist with management. Serological tests to identify viral causes are often not undertaken in self-limiting disease. If there is reason to suspect a connective tissue disease, other tests to identify the disorder can be performed.

Management in this case will be supportive. Monitoring for complications of myocarditis such as heart failure, conduction abnormalities, or rarely tamponade from a pericardial effusion is required in the immediate term. Long-term complications include a dilated cardiomyopathy with chronic heart failure.

 KEY POINTS

1. Myocarditis is uncommon but occurs in younger individuals and is most often due to a viral cause.
2. Acute myocarditis can mimic an acute myocardial infarction, and complications can include heart failure and conduction abnormalities.

CASE 70: DETERIORATING RENAL FUNCTION

History

A 73-year-old woman has been admitted with *Escherichia coli* bacteraemia secondary to pyelo-nephritis. Her history includes type 2 diabetes, hypertension, obesity, and osteoarthritis. She is taking a multitude of drugs: metformin 1 g twice daily; Levemir 16 units once daily; cande-sartan 32 mg once daily; paracetamol 1 g four times a day; spironolactone 12.5 mg once daily; and atorvastatin 10 mg once daily.

Initial Treatment

Candesartan was stopped on admission owing to her low blood pressure. She received a 7-day course of gentamicin and had a good clinical response. The investigation results were obtained on admission and on day 7 after admission.

INVESTIGATIONS

		Normal range
On admission		
Sodium	137	135–145 mmol/L
Potassium	3.8	3.5–5.0 mmol/L
Urea	7	3.0–7.0 mmol/L
Creatinine	120	60–110 µmol/L
Urine dipstick	Blood 2+, protein negative, nitrites positive, leu 2+	
Day 7 after admission		
Sodium	140	135–145 mmol/L
Potassium	6.0	3.5–5.0 mmol/L
Urea	35	3.0–7.0 mmol/L
Creatinine	300	60–110 µmol/L
Urine dipstick	Blood, protein, nitrites, leu all negative	

QUESTIONS

1. What are the possible causes of her change in urea and electrolyte results?
2. How would you manage this patient?

ANSWERS

The blood results are highly suggestive of an acute kidney injury (AKI). This is defined by any functional, structural, or markers of kidney damage occurring in the previous 3 months. AKI is one of a few classifications for acute renal failure—a historical term used to describe this condition.

AKI is divided into stages 1 to 3 and follows two criteria: (i) creatinine (Cr) and (ii) urine output (UO). Only one of the two criteria is needed for staging of AKI.

- Stage 1 = Cr increase >150%–200% from baseline or UO <0.5 mL/kg/h for more than 6 hours
- Stage 2 = Cr increase >200%–300% from baseline or UO <0.5 mL/kg/h for more than 12 hours
- Stage 3 = Cr increase >300% or Cr >350 μmol/L with acute rise of Cr >45 μmol/L or on renal replacement therapy or UO <0.3 mL/kg/h for 12 hours or anuria for 12 hours

Mortality rate increases with more advanced stages of AKI.

The initial management of AKI is to look for the underlying cause(s) and to reverse the immediate life-threatening complication associated with AKI. The causes of AKI are classified into:

- Pre-renal (hypotension, hypovolaemia, renovascular disease)
- Renal parenchymal (acute tubular necrosis, vasculitis, glomerular disorders, or tubulointerstitial disorders)
- Post-renal (urine outflow obstruction)

While the aetiology is being investigated it is important to review the patient's intravascular volume status (i.e. intravascular fluid depletion or fluid overload) and potassium level. These are potentially lethal associated conditions that must be dealt with urgently.

The approach for any AKI patient should include the following:

- Look for a history of systemic disorders that may contribute to current AKI (e.g. vascular diseases, diabetes, rheumatological disorders, myeloma, sepsis).
- Examine volume status and decide whether volume replacement or diuresis is needed. Careful charting of fluid balance is important to monitor treatment response and to set therapeutic goals.
- Examine for palpable bladder/enlarged prostate and loin pain. It is important to insert a urinary catheter to exclude bladder outflow obstruction.
- Measure electrolytes and obtain an arterial/venous blood gas to review potassium and bicarbonate levels. Acidaemia often worsens hyperkalaemia, and oral/intravenous sodium bicarbonate may sometimes be considered. A 12-lead ECG is needed to look for associated arrhythmia, especially when hyperkalaemia is present.
- Unless the patient is anuric, it is imperative to obtain a urine sample for dipstick, microbiology sampling, and cytological assessment. 'Bland' urine dipstick (all negative results) is highly suggestive of pre-renal AKI and acute tubular necrosis (ATN). Other rarer causes of bland urine are scleroderma, atherosclerotic emboli, and tubulointerstitial disorders. Blood on dipstick may suggest glomerulonephritis, vasculitis, thrombotic microangiopathy, haemoglobinuria, myoglobinuria, or trauma. Heavy proteinuria may be suggestive of nephrotic syndrome. Presence of white cells is suggestive of urinary tract infection or acute interstitial nephritis (eosinophils). Crystals found on urine examination may suggest urate nephropathy or drug-induced nephropathy (e.g. ethylene glycol/acyclovir). Urinary sodium and osmolality can

sometimes help differentiate pre-renal AKI from ATN, but in practice it is often difficult due to concurrent diuretic therapy.
- Perform urgent ultrasound of the renal tract to exclude urinary tract obstruction, examine for asymmetrical kidney size secondary to ischaemic nephropathy, and look for evidence of atrophic kidneys, which is highly suggestive of advanced chronic kidney disease (an exception is diabetic nephropathy, which retains 'normal' size kidneys).
- Look for evidence of chronic anaemia, hyperphosphataemia, or hypocalcaemia, which may suggest prior chronic kidney disease.
- Review recent drug histories carefully and stop all nephrotoxins. Also look for recent prescription of radiological contrast (weeks).
- In selected cases it may be important to request a liver function test (low albumin of nephrotic syndrome or hepatorenal syndrome); creatine kinase; urate (tumour lysis syndrome); lactate (hypoperfusion); prostate-specific antigen; antinuclear antibody; antineutrophil cytoplasmic antibody; rheumatoid factor; complement level; cryoglobulin level; hepatitis B and C serology; serum immunoglobulins; and serum protein electrophoresis (myeloma). All systemic disorders may lead to kidney disease.

When to start, which modality to use, and when to stop renal replacement therapy (haemodialysis or haemofiltration or both) are often debated. The emergency indications are (i) refractory or rapidly worsening hyperkalaemia and (ii) diuresis-resistant acute pulmonary oedema. Other indications for dialysis are (i) intractable metabolic acidosis (pH <7.1), (ii) uraemic pericarditis/encephalopathy, (iii) poison removal (e.g. lithium), and (iv) hyperthermia.

In the given scenario the two possible causes are ATN secondary to recent severe sepsis and/or gentamicin therapy. Gentamicin is an aminoglycoside antibiotic with a narrow therapeutic range. Aminoglycoside toxicity most commonly manifests as ototoxicity and nephrotoxicity, which is dose-dependent. The risk is related to the trough concentration rather than the peak concentration, so careful daily serum concentration monitoring is important. Studies suggest once-daily dosing of gentamicin is associated with less nephrotoxicity without affecting its bactericidal efficacy, so it is the more commonly used regimen. Often aminoglycosides can cause renal failure, and the accumulated level of drugs can further exacerbate this.

Gentamicin nephrotoxicity usually presents 7 days after initiation of therapy. It may also occur even after therapy is stopped. In most cases it is reversible upon aminoglycoside withdrawal. Risk factors include severe intercurrent illness, history of chronic kidney disease, diabetes, use of iodine-based radiological contrast, and concurrent use of potentially nephrotoxic drugs (e.g. non-steroidal anti-inflammatory drugs).

Gentamicin is dosed by *ideal* body weight (not actual body weight), and the daily maximum dose is 450 mg. A lower dose is often used in patients at risk of aminoglycoside nephropathy.

Other management considerations include stopping metformin, as it is excreted unchanged in urine, and data suggest that Cr >150 μmol/L is the threshold for withholding metformin, as it increases the risk of lactic acidosis. Spironolactone is a potassium-sparing diuretic and is best avoided in AKI also.

 KEY POINTS

1. Be familiar with the investigation and treatment of AKI.
2. Drugs can cause AKI, so a thorough drug history should be taken.
3. The renal drug handling changes with alteration in renal function, so frequent reviews are needed to avoid toxicity.

CASE 71: PETECHIAL RASH AND LOSS OF CONSCIOUSNESS

History

A 35-year-old man with Down's syndrome has been brought to the emergency department. He was difficult to arouse and appeared confused. His parents say that he has been very lethargic lately. Last night, he complained of a sore throat, headache, and nausea and vomiting.

Examination

This man looks unwell. Shortly after arrival, he had a tonic-clonic seizure which self-terminated in 1 minute. There is petechial rash, especially on pressure-dependent areas. His neck is stiff, and there are several palpable cervical lymph nodes. In the mouth, small ulcers are noted. Capillary refill is 3 seconds with cold peripheries. The rest of the cardiorespiratory examination is unremarkable. There is hepatosplenomegaly on abdominal palpation. His Glasgow Coma Scale score is E2/V3/M4. His tone is normal, but there is positive Babinski's sign bilaterally. Pupillary examination is difficult to conduct, but they are equal and reactive to light. Observations: temperature 38.5 °C, heart rate 112 beats/min, respiratory rate 32/min, blood pressure 90/60 mmHg, SpO_2 97% on room air.

INVESTIGATIONS

White cells	52.0
Neutrophils	0.4
Haemoglobin	6.8
Platelets	12
Sodium	135
Potassium	3.5
Urea	10
Creatinine	180
C-reactive protein	121
Bilirubin	35
Alanine aminotransferase	70
Alkaline phosphatase	156
Albumin	25
INR	1.9
D-dimer	5.2
Fibrinogen	0.7
Blood film	Presence of leukaemic lymphoblasts and schistocytes
Arterial blood gas on room air:	
pH	7.28
pO_2	10.0
pCO_2	3.0
Lactate	5.0
HCO_3	18

QUESTIONS

1. What is the cause of the critical illness?
2. What are the main laboratory abnormalities in the full blood count and clotting?
3. What should be the initial management plan?

DOI: 10.1201/9781003241171-71

ANSWERS

This man is critically unwell. He presents with clinical features of meningococcal sepsis with worrying signs of rapid clinical deterioration. Treatment should be started without delay.

The full blood count has an extremely high white cell count but neutropenia. The blood film confirmed the presence of leukaemic lymphoblasts that is suggestive of acute lymphocytic leukaemia. However, this requires a bone marrow aspiration and biopsy to confirm the diagnosis. Patients with Down's syndrome are predisposed to leukaemia, but they predominately present in their childhood. Despite the high white cell count, the cells have defective immune function, and the neutrophil production is suppressed. Therefore, patients are at risk of severe infection.

This man also has thrombocytopenia, low fibrinogen level, and raised INR and D-dimer. Although the thrombocytopenia could be in part due to bone marrow infiltration by lymphoblasts, taken together, this is due to consumption coagulopathy or disseminated intravascular coagulation (DIC). The presence of schistocytes, which are fragments of red cells, is also supportive of this. The clotting mechanisms in DIC are activated (raised D-dimer), and small thrombi form in the blood vessels, causing ischaemia. These clots consume large numbers of platelets and clotting factors (low fibrinogen), thus also causing abnormal bleeding. In this context the DIC is most likely due to meningococcal sepsis. The treatment of DIC can be complex, as it often occurs in the context of critically unwell patients. Support with blood products forms the mainstay of treatment in DIC (platelets, cryoprecipitate, and fresh frozen plasma). The anaemia is likely due to bone marrow infiltration by lymphoblasts and DIC.

The patient should be nursed in the recovery position with high-flow oxygen and monitored in a high-dependency area. Establish intravenous access if not already done so and have lorazepam ready in case he develops further seizures. His blood glucose should also be checked. In the context of critical illness and clotting abnormalities, lumbar puncture is contraindicated. Instead, the initial focus is on rapidly resuscitating his septic shock and DIC. Antibiotics covering meningococcal sepsis and neutropenia should be given, ideally before blood culture, but this should not delay the treatment. An early referral to intensive care is needed for airway management and transfer to critical care. As a biomarker, high lactate is closely correlated with the need for critical care admissions and mortality. A retrospective analysis suggests that even a 'normal' lactate from above 0.75 is correlated with mortality and poor outcome during a hospital admission. The metabolic acidosis is due to hyperlactataemia and acute kidney injury. His fluid resuscitation will include both crystalloids and blood products initially. High levels of blood products are probably needed to support bone marrow infiltration and DIC. The fluid status should be closely monitored, and vasopressors are most likely to be required.

🔑 KEY POINTS

1. Acute leukaemia may present the first time acutely as a medical emergency. The mortality rate is high in these circumstances.
2. Meningococcal sepsis is an important diagnosis not to miss, as clinical deterioration is fast and mortality is high. Prompt institution of antibiotics is essential, and lumbar puncture is not necessary. Meningococcal sepsis is a notifiable disease in the United Kingdom.

CASE 72: WHEEZE AND PRODUCTIVE COUGH

History

A 20-year-old woman has presented with severe shortness of breath associated with wheeze and productive cough. She was diagnosed with asthma at age 10 years. Until a year ago she had never been admitted to hospital, but since then she has been admitted three times with asthma exacerbations. She also complains of a chronic productive cough with large quantities of thick, dark sputum that is hard to expectorate. There is no other medical history, including sinusitis. She has never smoked. There is no travel history. She is taking a salbutamol inhaler, 2 puffs four times daily; Seretide 250, 2 puffs twice daily; and montelukast, 10 mg once daily.

Examination

This woman has pursed lip breathing, and she finds it difficult to complete a sentence in one breath. There is no clubbing or lymphadenopathy, peripheral oedema, or rash. Jugular venous pressure (JVP) is not raised. Her chest wall is overexpanded and chest expansion reduced but equal on both sides, and her trachea is central. There are coarse inspiratory crackles bilaterally in the mid-zones and polyphonic expiratory wheezes throughout her chest. Observations: temperature 37.9°C, heart rate 120 beats/min, respiratory rate 28/min, SpO_2 93% on room air.

🔍 INVESTIGATIONS

White cells	8.1
Neutrophils	5.0
Lymphocytes	0.9
Eosinophils	2.2
Haemoglobin	12.0
Platelets	188
C-reactive protein	24
Urine	Protein 1+ only
PEFR	100 L/min (best PEFR = 200L/min)

Arterial blood gas on room air:

pH	7.48
pO_2	8.9
pCO_2	3.2
Lactate	2.0
HCO_3	24
Base excess	0

Chest x-ray shows upper and middle lobe infiltrates and thickened bronchial wall markings.

❓ QUESTIONS

1. What is the acute diagnosis? What should be the initial management plan?
2. What is the likely cause for the worsening of asthma control in the last 12 months?

ANSWERS

This woman presents with an acute severe asthma attack. It is important to establish background asthma control, treatment plan, adherence, precipitating factors to current presentation, and red flags, e.g. any history of critical care admissions. The British guideline on the management of asthma (2019) defines the severity of an acute asthma attack (moderate vs. acute severe vs. life-threatening asthma) according to several parameters: best/predicted peak expiratory flow rate, SpO_2, respiratory rate, heart rate, paO_2 and $paCO_2$, degree of respiratory effort (e.g. ability to complete a sentence), and signs of exhaustion. The management plan is dependent on the severity at presentation and the outcome of the interval reassessments. All initial treatments of severe/life-threatening attacks involve a beta₂-agonist, usually salbutamol 5 mg delivered by oxygen-driven nebuliser, and steroids (oral prednisolone 40 to 50 mg or intravenous hydrocortisone 100 mg). Repeated salbutamol and/or ipratropium and intravenous magnesium may also be required. Any features of life-threatening asthma will require early input from critical care.

The chest x-ray shows infiltrates and thickened bronchial wall markings that are not typical of asthma. The history of chronic productive cough and inspiratory crackles on examination and the chest x-ray findings are more in keeping with bronchiectasis. This can be confirmed by high-resolution CT scan. Furthermore, there is a moderately raised eosinophilia, which cannot be explained by asthma alone, as it usually causes a mild eosinophilia ($<1.5 \times 10^9$/L) only. Several disorders can cause blood eosinophilia and lung disease. In the history, there is a lack of recent change in drug history or travel history to suggest drug-induced or parasitic causes. The other possible causes are allergic bronchopulmonary aspergillosis (ABPA), eosinophilic granulomatosis with polyangiitis (previously Churg-Strauss syndrome), chronic eosinophilic pneumonia, and hypereosinophilic syndrome.

ABPA is due to an abnormal immune response to *Aspergillus* spores. *Aspergillus* is a fungus that is ubiquitous and is present in the sputum of most people. Atopic patients develop immunoglobulin E (IgE) and immunoglobulin G (IgG) against *Aspergillus* spores, leading to an allergic response that in turn causes bronchial obstruction with dark mucus plugs, haemoptysis, malaise, and fever. ABPA can lead to recurrent chest infections, bronchiectasis, and pulmonary fibrosis. Diagnosis of ABPA is established by skin prick testing demonstrating an immediate skin sensitivity to *Aspergillus*, raised total serum IgE (>417 kilounits/L), and the presence of *Aspergillus*-specific IgE/IgG. CT chest can identify the presence and extent of bronchiectasis or pulmonary fibrosis. Chronic eosinophilic pneumonia can present like ABPA, but the immunology tests for *Aspergillus* will be negative. In this case there is a lack of features to suggest eosinophilic granulomatosis with polyangiitis. The typical features are sinusitis, peripheral neuropathy, palpable purpura, and positive antineutrophil cytoplasmic antibodies. Hypereosinophilic syndrome is characterised by eosinophil infiltration to multiple organs, and patients tend to present with a variety of symptoms, including angioedema, myocarditis, cardiomyopathy, encephalopathy, interstitial lung disease, pleural effusions, arterial and venous thromboembolism, encephalopathy, peripheral neuropathy, gastritis, hepatosplenomegaly, and arthropathy.

Given the history of this patient, it is important to establish whether she has ABPA and bronchiectasis. Once the diagnosis of ABPA is established, the mainstay treatment is with oral steroids daily, which are weaned off over a period of 8 weeks. The antifungal itraconazole is an adjunct in reducing exacerbations of ABPA. Serum IgE is a useful marker for monitoring response and detecting exacerbation. Patients should be counselled to avoid high exposures to *Aspergillus*, which are typically in dead and decaying organic matter such as compost piles. Any damp and water damage in the patient's home should be repaired to avoid exposure to mould.

 KEY POINTS

1. Worsening asthma symptoms in previously well-controlled asthmatic patients should prompt investigation of the underlying cause.
2. Acute asthma attack is a common medical emergency that should be dealt with promptly. National guidelines are available to guide management decisions.

CASE 73: FLU-LIKE ILLNESS AND GENERALISED WEAKNESS

History

A 67-year-old man attends the emergency department complaining of a 1-day history of productive cough with purulent sputum. In the last month, he has developed dizziness, nausea, anorexia, and progressive generalised weakness. His medical history includes hypertension and metastatic adenocarcinoma of the lung. He is an ex-smoker, and he does not drink alcohol or use herbal or recreational drugs. He has not travelled abroad in the last 10 years. His drug history includes amlodipine and pembrolizumab.

Examination

This man looks unwell—dehydrated with dry lips and reduced skin turgor. A 30 mmHg postural hypotension is noted. His jugular venous pulse (JVP) is not visible in the recumbent position. Heart sounds are normal. Chest examination shows inspiratory crackles on the right middle zone on auscultation. Abdominal and neurological examinations were unremarkable. Observations: temperature 38.3°C, heart rate 120 beats/min, blood pressure 100/60 mmHg, respiratory rate 28/min, SpO_2 92% on room air.

🔍 INVESTIGATIONS

	Normal range
White cells	15.2
Neutrophils	11.4
Haemoglobin	11.0
Platelets	168
Sodium	110
Potassium	5.5
Urea	10
Creatinine	128
Corrected calcium	2.25
Urate	317
C-reactive protein	56
Glucose	3.0

Arterial blood gas sample on room air:

pH	7.31
pO_2	8.2
pCO_2	3.0
Lactate	2.1
HCO_3	16 22–26 mmol/L
Base excess	−3 −3 to +3 mmol/L

12-lead ECG: Sinus tachycardia.

Chest x-ray	Right hilar mass with new right-sided consolidation and air bronchogram in the mid-zone.

❓ QUESTIONS

1. What is the diagnosis of this man's presentation?
2. How would you manage this patient in an acute general medical setting?

DOI: 10.1201/9781003241171-73

ANSWERS

This man is clearly very unwell. He has clinical signs of severe intravascular fluid deficit and pneumonia. The laboratory investigations show a severe hyponatraemia, hyperkalaemia, acute kidney injury, hypoglycaemia, metabolic acidosis with respiratory compensation, and raised inflammatory markers. The combined metabolic and electrolyte derangements (hyponatraemia, hyperkalaemia, metabolic acidosis, and hypoglycaemia) is suggestive of an underlying adrenal insufficiency.

In the first instance, this man should be nursed and fully monitored in a high-dependency area. Oxygen should be given to target an oxygen saturation of at least 94%. Multiple large-bore intravenous accesses should be established as soon as possible to manage the hypovolaemia and electrolyte disturbance, in particular the hyponatraemia. Fluid balance and frequent fluid status assessments are required, and a urinary catheter may be needed to monitor urine output. A bolus of fluid should be given as a fluid challenge as soon as possible. Interval laboratory samples should be taken to track changes in sodium, potassium, lactate, glucose, and metabolic acidosis. Glucose replacement should be administered with care to prevention exacerbation of hyponatraemia. Antibiotics for the treatment of community-acquired pneumonia should be initiated without delay.

Although it is important to obtain a 9 am plasma adrenocorticotropic hormone (ACTH) and cortisol level and to perform a short ACTH stimulation test to confirm adrenal insufficiency, patients are often too unwell, and these tests must not delay the administration of fluid and steroids (e.g. hydrocortisone) immediately. If possible, a random sample of cortisol and ACTH should be taken before steroid therapy. High-dose steroid treatment in adrenal crisis has sufficient mineralocorticoid activity, and fludrocortisone can be introduced later if required. In this case, the adrenal insufficiency is likely to be due to pembrolizumab or adrenal metastasis. Pembrolizumab is an immunotherapy acting as an immune checkpoint inhibitor by binding to the programmed cell death-1 (PD-1) receptor that is expressed by all T cells during activation. PD-1 is essential to the central and peripheral T-cell tolerance, aiding in the protection of self-tissues from autoimmune responses. The blocking of PD-1 interaction with its ligand lifts this immune checkpoint and increases T cells anti-tumour response in susceptible tumours. Immune checkpoint inhibitors have increasingly diverse indications as first-line treatment for multiple cancers. One of the most important groups of adverse reaction is the 'on-target, off tumour toxicities' causing inflammation in other organ systems—immune-related pneumonitis, colitis, hepatitis, skin reactions, and endocrinopathies (thyroid, pituitary, and adrenal glands). In this case, it is important to obtain oncology and endocrinology inputs. The pembrolizumab should be withheld for now, and the lung cancer should be re-evaluated when he is stabilised.

🔑 KEY POINTS

1. The presenting symptoms of adrenal insufficiency are non-specific, so a high index of suspicion is needed to make the diagnosis.
2. It is ideal to take a 9 am cortisol blood sample and perform a Synacthen test to make the diagnosis of adrenal insufficiency prior to instigating steroid treatment. However, in an acute medical emergency, empirical steroids should be given as a priority without delay.

CASE 74: FEVER AND A MURMUR

History

A 45-year-old man presented with progressive breathlessness and fever for last 2–3 weeks. His past medical history was unremarkable. Observations showed a temp of 38.2°C, HR 92 bpm, BP 123/58 mmHg, RR 18 breaths/min, oxygen saturations 94% on room air. On examination, he was noted to have a murmur and basal lung crepitations. His JVP was also elevated. No other abnormalities were noted on physical examination. Further enquiry revealed he had attended the dentist about a month ago. There was no foreign travel or other unwell members of his immediate family. On systems review he had no cough or gastrointestinal (GI) disturbance. There were no joint problems or skin rashes.

His chest x-ray (CXR) showed bilateral perihilar pulmonary shadowing and upper lobe blood diversion.

A bedside echo was performed and identified aortic regurgitation and a mobile mass 1 cm × 2 cm on one of the aortic cusps.

Blood tests showed:

Blood test	Result	Normal range
White cells	9.0	$4–11 \times 109/L$
Haemoglobin	12.0	13–18 g/dL
Platelets	350	$150–400 \times 109/L$
Sodium	135	135–145 mmol/L
Potassium	3.6	3.5–5.0 mmol/L
Urea	5.0	3.0–7.0 mmol/L
Creatinine	60	60–110 umol/L
CRP	140	<5 mg/L

> **? QUESTIONS**
> 1. What is the diagnosis?
> 2. How is this condition treated?

ANSWERS

1. The presentation is in keeping with infective endocarditis of the aortic valve complicated by aortic regurgitation and pulmonary oedema. The patient's history of a previous dental procedure may be associated with the development of infective endocarditis, but it is more likely to be associated in higher-risk individuals, e.g. patients with previous infective endocarditis, prosthetic heart valves, or uncorrected congenital cyanotic heart disease. Indeed, it is currently preferred practice to administer prophylactic antibiotics to such high-risk patients undergoing high-risk dental procedures, such as any manipulation of the gingival or periapical region or oral mucosal perforation like scaling and root canal work. Immediate management in this case is to treat the pulmonary oedema and obtain blood cultures urgently with a view to commencing broad-spectrum antibiotics. Close monitoring for haemodynamic compromise is required on a high-dependency unit or coronary care unit. Complications can arise quickly, including acute pulmonary oedema, heart block from aortic root abscess formation, fistulas and perforations, myocardial infarction, or strokes from embolic events.

   Diagnosis is based on the use of the Modified Dukes Criteria, but a high index of suspicion is required in any patient with a fever of unknown cause. The most common organisms are oral *Streptococcus* species and *Staphylococcus* from skin commensals. Immunocompromised patients may have other causative organisms, including fungal.

2. The general management of infective endocarditis is to treat the infection and prevent or manage complications. Infective endocarditis has a high mortality and requires a multi-disciplinary endocarditis team to manage appropriately, consisting of a cardiology, microbiology, and cardiothoracic surgical team. Prolonged courses of antibiotics targeted to the causative organism is required, with longer duration for prosthetic valves over native valves. Ideally, rendering the patient sterile and free of infection before any surgical intervention, if required, to repair or replace damaged valves is preferred. However, early intervention may be required if there are complications including haemodynamic compromise from acute valve regurgitation causing heart failure, embolic events, or the development of aortic root abscess complications.

   Most patients present with a fever (90%) with the finding of a heart murmur in up to 85% of patients. Embolic complications occur in up to 25% at presentation and should be looked for when investigating a patient with a fever and a murmur. Investigations could include brain MRI or CT to look for embolism in the cerebral hemispheres. Thorough bedside examination looking for vascular and immunological phenomena of infective endocarditis is useful but may not be present (e.g. splinter haemorrhages, Roth spots, Janeway lesions, and Osler's nodes). The main method of diagnosis remains echocardiography alongside microbiological evidence of typical organisms associated with endocarditis. In particular circumstances if a vegetation is not obvious on transthoracic echocardiography, a transoesophageal echocardiogram to visualise the valve apparatus more clearly or whole-body imaging (e.g. CT-PET [positron emission tomography]) can be used in cases of prosthetic valves or if index of suspicion is high.

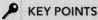

KEY POINTS

1. Infective endocarditis should be considered in any patient with an unexplained fever and a heart murmur.
2. Management of infective endocarditis requires a multi-disciplinary team to consider antibiotic choice and duration and the requirement for and timing of surgical intervention.

CASE 75: WHEEZE AND SHORTNESS OF BREATH

History

A 38-year-old man has presented to the emergency department with shortness of breath and wheeze. On arrival he was in extremis and unable to complete a full sentence. He was discharged from the hospital 1 week ago after acute severe exacerbation of chronic obstructive pulmonary disease (COPD), first diagnosed 3 years ago. This is his third casualty attendance over the past 12 months. He smokes five cigarettes a day. He is now awaiting investigation for deranged liver function tests. His father died of a chest disease in his 30s. He is taking salbutamol inhaler, tiotropium inhaler, budesonide/formoterol inhaler, carbocisteine, and Uniphyllin Continus.

Examination

This man is visibly dyspnoeic with a respiratory rate of 32/min and using accessory muscles. His trachea is central, chest is hyperexpanded and the degree of expansion is poor but equal, and auscultation reveals widespread expiratory wheeze but no clinical sign of consolidation. Observations: heart rate 130 beats/min, blood pressure 130/80 mmHg, SpO_2 87% on room air, FiO_2 0.24.

🔍 INVESTIGATIONS

White cells	15.0
Haemoglobin	13.0
Platelets	150
Sodium	140
Potassium	3.2
Urea	7.1
Creatinine	100
C-reactive protein	10
Bilirubin	62
Aspartate aminotransferase	138
Alkaline phosphatase	215
Albumin	31
INR	1.2
Arterial blood gas on FiO_2 0.24:	
pH	7.23
pO_2	6.7
pCO^2	8.2
Lactate	2.3
HCO_3	29
Chest x-ray	Hyperinflated lung fields. No pneumothorax or consolidation.

❓ QUESTIONS

1. What are the differential diagnoses?
2. What is the appropriate initial management?
3. What is the unifying diagnosis, and how would you confirm it?

ANSWERS

The main differential diagnoses for this man's acute shortness of breath are acute exacerbation of COPD and pulmonary embolism. The chest x-ray finding did not show evidence of acute pulmonary oedema, pneumothorax, or pneumonia. The clinical findings are more in keeping with an acute exacerbation of COPD.

This man presents with type 2 respiratory failure, and the arterial blood gas results on 24% of supplemental oxygen showed a significant hypoxia with respiratory acidosis and partially compensated metabolic alkalosis. His very high respiratory rate and arterial blood gas results are worrying and require referral to critical care whilst treatment is ongoing. As with all acutely unwell patients, airway, breathing, and circulation should be managed accordingly, and the patient should be nursed in a high-dependency area, with cardiorespiratory monitoring. Venous access should be established, and a 12-lead ECG should be taken. It is important to establish background COPD control, co-morbidities, treatment plan, adherence, precipitating factors to current presentation, and red flags, e.g. any history of critical care admissions.

The definition and treatment of acute exacerbation of COPD are summarised by the National Institute for Health and Care Excellence (NICE) guideline NG115. The pharmacological management in this case includes appropriate oxygen therapy, nebulised bronchodilators (β2 agonists, anticholinergics, and theophyllines), steroids, and antibiotics. The delivery gas (oxygen vs. medical air) for the nebuliser should be specified. Patients taking oral theophylline therapy should have the theophylline level measured at admission to determine whether it is at a subtherapeutic or toxic level. This is particularly important if intravenous theophylline therapy is considered. Oxygen is a drug, and it should be given correctly by selecting an appropriate delivery device. The British Thoracic Society guideline for oxygen use in adults in health care and emergency settings (2017) provides comprehensive guidance on this. In the context of type 2 respiratory failure, a fixed performance device should be selected (e.g. Venturi device) to reduce the risk of carbon dioxide narcosis. The key is to repeat clinical assessment frequently in the acute setting. Repeat arterial blood gas (preferably with local anaesthesia in the absence of arterial catheter) should be conducted 30–60 minutes after any changes to oxygen treatment. The titration should consider the patient's previous and latest arterial blood gas results and current respiratory effort and rate. Non-invasive ventilation in the form of bilevel positive airway pressure (BIPAP) or mechanical ventilation is likely to be required in this case if the patient does not rapidly respond to bronchodilator treatment. The British Thoracic Society guideline for the ventilatory management of acute hypercapnic respiratory failure in adults (2016) provides detailed guidance on this. Bronchodilators could be delivered via a BIPAP device concurrently, which is useful in the treatment of acute exacerbation of COPD.

This man was diagnosed with COPD at a very young age. It may be appropriate to review his case histories and previous lung function tests, chest imaging, and bronchodilator reversibility tests to ensure this patient is not suffering from asthma rather than COPD. If COPD is confirmed, then further investigation should be considered. In the setting of a positive family history of early death due to chest disease and a history of deranged liver function tests, α1-antitrypsin deficiency (A1AD) should be excluded.

A1AD is one of the most common genetic disorders, with an autosomal dominant inheritance. The protease inhibitor enzyme α1-antitrypsin is responsible for neutralising neutrophil elastase, and the deficiency in α1-antitrypsin leads to damage to the lungs and the liver. There are a large number of possible genotypes and phenotypes, so the expression of α1-antitrypsin is variable even for patients from the same family. The severity of organ damage is in part determined by environmental factors such as smoking and dust exposure; thus it is paramount to encourage smoking cessation. Presentation (if not diagnosed through family screening) is often at the third or fourth decade with emphysematous lung changes out of proportion to smoking history. The emphysematous changes are predominately in the lower zones, but it can affect all lung fields. Bronchiectasis may also occur. Only a proportion of homozygous A1AD cases develop cirrhosis, but some patients may present this way in childhood or in later adulthood, especially those who never smoked. Other complications of A1AD include relapsing panniculitis and granulomatosis with polyangiitis. Serum α1-antitrypsin level, genotyping, and phenotyping are required to confirm the diagnosis of A1AD. Treatment of A1AD is similar to standard COPD therapy, with smoking cessation particularly emphasised. α1-antitrypsin replacement is not recommended by NICE, as the clinical benefit is currently uncertain. Lung and/or liver transplant may be options for some patients. A1AD patients should be managed at a specialist centre, and their family should be offered genetic counselling.

🔑 KEY POINTS

1. Acute exacerbation of COPD is a common acute medical emergency that should be recognised and treated promptly.
2. A1AD is one of the most commonly inherited genetic disorders. Smoking cessation is the key in halting its lung manifestations.

CASE 76: RED EYES AND SIGHT IMPAIRMENT

History

A 20-year-old man of Japanese descent attends the emergency department with a 2-day history of bilateral painful red eyes with blurred vision and photophobia. In the past year, he had one episode of deep vein thrombosis in his left leg and recurrent oral and genital ulcers over the scrotum. His acne has also been worsening in the last few months, and it is now extending to his back and his limbs. There is no significant sexual history of note.

Examination

There are bilateral ciliary and conjunctival injection. The pupils are small and react to light sluggishly. Ophthalmoscopy is not possible owing to discomfort in bright light. The patient has a visual acuity of 6/9 bilaterally. There is no evidence of lymphadenopathy, but there are multiple aphthous ulcers in the oral cavity. There are also multiple tender nodules over the shins bilaterally, and his right knee joint has minimal effusion and limited movements. His cardiorespiratory, abdominal, and neurological examinations are unremarkable.

🔍 INVESTIGATIONS

White cells	9.0
Haemoglobin	11.7
Platelets	300
Sodium	136
Potassium	3.9
Urea	3.7
Creatinine	85
C-reactive protein	56
Rheumatoid factor	Negative
Antinuclear antibodies	Negative
Antineutrophil cytoplasmic antibodies	Negative

❓ QUESTIONS

1. How would you manage this man's red eyes?
2. What is the unifying diagnosis of this man's condition?

DOI: 10.1201/9781003241171-76

ANSWERS

This man presents with acute bilateral painful red eyes associated with blurred vision and photophobia. This is an ophthalmic emergency requiring urgent ophthalmology input to confirm the diagnosis. The main differential diagnoses are uveitis, keratitis, and glaucoma. In this case the ophthalmologist was able to confirm anterior uveitis as the cause following a slit lamp examination performed with mydriatics. Anterior uveitis tends to affect one eye at presentation, but bilateral disease can occur. The major concern here is the potential threat to his vision. Topical steroids and mydriatics should be started with close follow-up of his condition. Systemic immunosuppressive drugs may be required in severe cases. Anterior uveitis is associated with several systemic conditions, and these should be enquired:

- Seronegative arthropathies such as ankylosing spondylitis
- Behçet's syndrome
- Psoriasis
- Reactive arthritis
- Inflammatory bowel disease
- Sarcoidosis
- Infection—toxoplasmosis, herpes simplex, varicella zoster virus, and tuberculosis

The collection of features, including orogenital ulcers, monoarthritis, anterior uveitis, erythema nodosum, and history of venous thromboembolism, is highly suggestive of Behçet's syndrome. Other features include parenchymal lesions and vascular thrombosis of the central nervous system, ulcerations in the gastrointestinal tract that can present as bleeding or mimicking inflammatory bowel disease, and aneurysms, especially the pulmonary arteries. The multi-system nature of this illness is reflected by the underlying pathology as a systemic vasculitis. The prevalence of Behçet's syndrome is highest in Turkey, but patients from the 'Silk Road' territories, i.e. from the Middle East, Mediterranean to East Asia, are also disproportionally affected. The pathergy test is positive in 60% of patients, and it is a useful clinical diagnostic test for Behçet's syndrome. It is positive when indurations occur 1–2 days after a skin prick. The first-line treatment for the ulcers is topical corticosteroids. In refractory or more severe cases, systemic corticosteroids, colchicine, or another immunosuppressant such as azathioprine and thalidomide may be required. Other manifestations in the eye, gastrointestinal tract, vascular system, and central nervous system require systemic corticosteroids and immunosuppressants such as azathioprine or cyclophosphamide. Venous thrombosis is managed by immunosuppression and anticoagulation. Most patients enter remission over time, and lifelong treatment with immunosuppressants is not required.

🔑 KEY POINTS

1. It is important to recognise and establish the underlying cause of acute uveitis.
2. Acute uveitis is a sight-threatening condition that should be recognised and treated promptly.
3. Behçet's syndrome is a systemic vasculitis with a distinct pattern of clinical features.

CASE 77: SEVERE ABDOMINAL PAIN AND FEVER

History

A 69-year-old woman has presented to the emergency department with a 2-day history of severe right upper quadrant abdominal pain. This was colicky in nature initially but has now progressed to constant abdominal pain. Her pain is associated with dark urine, and her children noticed she had yellow discolouration on her skin and her eyes in the morning when they came to visit her. She also reports poor oral intake over the past week and has felt feverish with rigors since yesterday. She was previously fit and well.

Examination

This woman is icteric and looks unwell with reduced skin turgor and dry tongue. She feels cool to the touch up to her wrists and her ankles. There is no clubbing or lymphadenopathy. Her jugular venous pulse (JVP) cannot be seen, and her pulse volume is reduced. Capillary refill is 2 seconds. The cardiorespiratory examination is otherwise normal. There is tenderness in the upper abdomen with positive Murphy's sign. Bowel sounds are present. A rectal examination is unremarkable. Observations: temperature 39°C, heart rate 120 beats/min, blood pressure 98/57 mmHg, respiratory rate 28/min, SaO$_2$ 93% on room air.

🔍 INVESTIGATIONS

		Normal range
White cells	20.0	4–11 × 10⁹/L
Neutrophils	18.4	2–7 × 10⁹/L
Haemoglobin	12.8	13–18 g/dL
Platelets	180	150–400 × 10⁹/L
Sodium	135	135–145 mmol/L
Potassium	3.6	3.5–5.0 mmol/L
Urea	12	3.0–7.0 mmol/L
Creatinine	180	60–110 µmol/L
C-reactive protein	310	<5 mg/L
Amylase	300	20–110 IU/L
Bilirubin	80	5–25 µmol/L
Alanine aminotransferase	100	8–55 IU/L
Alkaline phosphatase	340	42–98 IU/L
Albumin	30	35–50 g/L
Gamma-glutamyl transpeptidase	111	8–78 IU/L
INR	1.8	0.9–1.1
Arterial blood gas on room air:		
pH	7.29	7.35–7.45
pO$_2$	11.0	9.3–13.3 kPa
pCO$_2$	3.2	4.7–6.0 kPa
Lactate	4.0	<2 mmol/L
HCO$_3$	18	22–26 mmol/L
Base excess	−4	−3 to +3 mmol/L

❓ QUESTIONS

1. What is the most likely diagnosis?
2. How would you manage this woman?

ANSWERS

Fever, jaundice, and right upper quadrant abdominal pain make up the Charcot's triad, which includes the main signs and symptoms of acute cholangitis. If a patient presents with Charcot's triad and altered mental status and shock, it is called Reynold's pentad. This woman has presented with Reynold's pentad and will require urgent resuscitation.

The most common cause of acute cholangitis is gallstone disease. Other causes are tumours (such as pancreatic cancer or cholangiocarcinoma) and strictures associated with previous biliary tree instrumentation. These processes lead to biliary tract outflow obstruction and bacterial infection. The most common bacteria are gram-negative organisms such as *Escherichia coli*, although enterococci and anaerobes could also be responsible.

The first step of this patient's resuscitation is to ensure she is fully monitored in a high-dependency area. Oxygen should be given to ensure SaO_2 of at least 94%. Intravenous access and blood cultures should be taken, and intravenous fluid and antibiotics should be given as soon as possible. A bolus fluid challenge should be delivered to ensure her mean arterial pressure (MAP) is above 65 mmHg. MAP is used as the resuscitation target, as it is more closely related to organ perfusion. This woman has evidence of acute kidney injury, so a urinary catheter should be inserted to monitor urine output. Reviewing clinical status frequently is very important in the resuscitation of any critically ill patient.

Part of the Surviving Sepsis guidelines (www.survivingsepsis.org) highlight the importance of 'source identification and control'. As acute cholangitis is caused by biliary obstruction, it is important to establish what is causing the blockage. An urgent ultrasound of the abdomen should be arranged to look for gallstones and a dilated common bile duct. In experienced hands, ultrasound of the biliary tree is the best modality in identifying gallstones. Another increasingly common modality to be used is magnetic resonance cholangiopancreatography (MRCP), which gives a clear image of the anatomy of the biliary tree and the pancreatic duct. Therapeutic endoscopic retrograde cholangiopancreatography (ERCP) is useful in relieving obstructing gallstones in the common bile duct and to insert stent(s) for malignant strictures to temporarily relieve biliary obstruction.

> **KEY POINTS**
>
> 1. Acute cholangitis carries a high mortality.
> 2. It is important to treat acute cholangitis promptly with antibiotics and control the source as appropriate.

CASE 78: RASH AND FLU-LIKE SYMPTOMS

History

A 42-year-old man has presented to his general practitioner (GP) with a 1-week history of flu-like symptoms, including general malaise, fever, headache, muscle aches, and joint pains. He notes that his joint pains have moved from one joint to another over the past week. He also complains of multiple rashes on his lower limbs, which started as papules and then evolved daily into large erythematous lesions with areas of paleness in the middle of these lesions. He has no medical history, and there has been no recent travel history abroad. He works as a gamekeeper on Exmoor.

Examination

There is a small area of cellulitis over the left calf. On the right lower leg there are multiple annular target-like erythematous rashes that are 8 cm in diameter. On the left knee there is a large, tender erythematous swelling, but no other joints are affected. The rest of the clinical examination is unremarkable. Observations: temperature 37.9°C, heart rate 100 beats/min, blood pressure 120/80 mmHg, SaO_2 100% on room air.

🔍 INVESTIGATIONS

		Normal range
White cells	22.0	$4\text{--}11 \times 10^9/L$
Haemoglobin	15.0	13–18 g/dL
Platelets	178	$150\text{--}400 \times 10^9/L$
Sodium	136	135–145 mmol/L
Potassium	4.2	3.5–5.0 mmol/L
Urea	7.6	3.0–7.0 mmol/L
Creatinine	89	60–110 µmol/L
INR	1.0	0.9–1.1

Left knee joint aspirate:	
Appearance	Straw-coloured with translucent clarity
Cell count	Presence of leucocytes (2000 cells/mm3)
ECG	Sinus tachycardia rate 102/min

❓ QUESTIONS

1. What is the likely diagnosis?
2. What is the appropriate management?

DOI: 10.1201/9781003241171-78

ANSWERS

The description is consistent with Lyme borreliosis, which is the most common human tick-borne zoonosis in the northern hemisphere. *Borrelia burgdorferi* is the most common type of spirochaete leading to Lyme disease in the UK. The transmitting vector is an ixodid tick, which normally feeds on large mammals and birds. Humans may be incidental hosts, and infection typically occurs at the nymphal stage of its life cycle.

Primary prevention through appropriate clothing and the use of skin insect repellents containing *N,N*-diethyl-meta-toluamide (DEET) may reduce the risk of Lyme disease. Regular body checking for tick bites is also important. Not all tick bites are infective, and antibiotic prophylaxis is not routinely recommended. Tick bite sufferers are normally advised to remove ticks with toothed tweezers and monitor for signs of erythema migrans (see later). Serological testing for asymptomatic individuals is also not recommended. The normal incubation period of Lyme is 1–2 weeks, and not all patients infected with *Borrelia* are symptomatic. In suspected cases of Lyme disease, it is usual to treat with antibiotics empirically; the recommended regimen in the UK is either amoxicillin or doxycycline. Serological testing is not always needed if the presentation is typical. The timing of serological testing is important, as most patients will be seropositive only 2–4 weeks after the onset of symptoms, and even then the testing is not 100% sensitive.

The presentation of Lyme disease varies greatly. Three-quarters of cases develop erythema migrans, with target-like erythematous lesions. These lesions may become chronic and develop into cellulitis-like lesions. Rarely, acrodermatitis chronica atrophicans—with chronic blue lesions—occurs, and it typically affects the extensor surfaces of limbs accompanied by peripheral neuropathy. Another rare skin manifestation, which typically occurs in cases outside Europe, is borrelial lymphocytoma—with plaque-like lesions mimicking cutaneous lymphoma.

Other manifestations occur in the nervous system (bilateral cranial nerve 7 palsies, subacute lymphocytic meningitis/encephalitis, subacute demyelinating and axonal sensory/motor neuropathy causing severe radicular nerve root pain, and mononeuritis multiplex), cardiovascular system (myocarditis, second-/third-degree heart block), and arthropathies, which typically affect large joints causing large swelling but surprisingly little accompanying pain. If left untreated, this arthropathy may become chronic.

> **🔑 KEY POINTS**
>
> 1. Lyme borreliosis can potentially have multi-system manifestations.
> 2. It is not always necessary to have a positive Lyme serology prior to initiation of treatment.

CASE 79: SUBSTANCE ABUSE AND AGITATION

History

A 40-year-old woman has been brought to the emergency department by her friends from the local nightclub. She is agitated, confused, and verbally aggressive. The friends report a fitting episode lasting 30 seconds en route to the hospital. They also say that she has taken "some pills". She refuses to cooperate with staff and says she wants to dance.

Examination

She will not agree to a full examination but cooperates enough for observations to be obtained: temperature 38°C, heart rate 130 beats/min (regular), blood pressure 170/130 mmHg, SpO_2 99% on room air. She is noted to have excessive diaphoresis and has grossly dilated pupils (size 5). There is no hyperreflexia or clonus.

? QUESTIONS

1. What are the differential diagnoses of this woman's presentation?
2. What is the appropriate management?

ANSWERS

This woman has acute recreational drug toxicity. Despite the difficulty in engaging with her, every effort should be made to take a focused history from the patient or collateral history to ascertain the type of substance exposed; the amount and route of administration; the time of the event; co-ingestion of other substances, e.g. alcohol; co-morbidities; drug history; and if appropriate, any administration of antidote or supportive treatment (e.g. naloxone, benzodiazepines). The information is helpful in predicting the likely effect of the poison(s) over time so that appropriate and timely treatment can be given. Beware of slang terms or street names describing recreational drugs, as the ingredients can vary considerably in different geographical regions and over time. For example 'ecstasy' can be methylenedioxymethamphetamine (MDMA) or benzylpiperazine or 'liquid ecstasy'/gamma-hydroxybutyrate (GHB). A 'drug screen' or 'toxicology screen' is rarely necessary in the acute setting. This is because the turnaround time for the results is 1–2 weeks, and it is not possible to screen for all possible toxins, so it does not alter the immediate management of the poisoned patient. In all cases the most important step is to identify the presenting toxidrome, which is a cluster of symptoms and signs that point to a particular group of poisons so that appropriate supportive treatment or antidotes can be provided. In the UK, the most common ones are anticholinergic, cholinergic, sedatives, opioids, sympathomimetics, and serotonin toxidromes. It is important to note that toxidromes may overlap, as some substances can cause more than one toxidrome, and co-ingestion of more than one substance is common. In this case, the agitation, mydriasis, excessive diaphoresis, hyperthermia, tachycardia, and hypertension rules out cholinergic (miosis, excessive secretions, bradycardia, and hypotension) or sedative/opiate (reduced consciousness, miosis, and hypotension) poisoning. The differential diagnoses are anticholinergics, sympathomimetics, or drugs that cause serotonin toxicity. Excessive diaphoresis is not in keeping with anticholinergic poisoning, as this usually causes dry eyes, dry mouth, and urinary retention. Therefore, the most likely toxidromes are sympathomimetic and/or drugs that can cause serotonin syndrome. In both toxidromes, the central characteristic is over-simulation of the central nervous system. Clinical features that are more specific to serotonin syndrome are spontaneous or inducible clonus and autonomic instability (e.g. variable heart rate and blood pressure).

As with most medical emergencies, the airway, breathing, and circulation (ABC) should be assessed and managed appropriately. Neurological examinations should be carried out to examine pupillary reflex and to look for clonus, hyperreflexia, and hypertonia. Blood glucose should be checked, especially with a history of seizure activity. Other investigations include electrocardiogram (for QRS interval prolongation due to sodium channel blockade and/or QT interval prolongation due to potassium channel blockade); blood test for renal function; creatine kinase; liver function tests; and calcium, bicarbonate, and chloride levels. The hyperthermia in this case is a sign of severe poisoning and a poor prognostic sign. The main aim of the treatment for both sympathomimetic and serotonin syndrome is to reduce central nervous system stimulation by sedation with benzodiazepines. Most symptoms will respond to benzodiazepine, but repeat doses may be required. Cooling with cold intravenous fluids and/or cool packs is an additional measure to aggressively control hyperthermia. Intravenous fluid is also useful for the initial treatment of hypotension and for rhabdomyolysis, but careful monitoring of electrolytes is required.

Further collateral history from this patient's friend confirms MDMA poisoning. MDMA is an amphetamine sympathomimetic with potential to cause serotonin syndrome. Important side effects specific to acute toxicity of this drug are cardiac arrhythmia (supraventricular or ventricular); hyponatraemia (secondary to excess water consumption and excess secretion of antidiuretic hormone); cerebral haemorrhage (secondary to severe hypertension); aortic dissection; myocardial infarction; mesenteric ischaemia; seizure; and a hyperthermic syndrome leading to acute kidney injury, disseminated intravascular coagulation, rhabdomyolysis, and hepatocellular necrosis. Tachycardia and hypertension usually resolve with benzodiazepines. Beta-blockers should be avoided, as they can cause unopposed vascular alpha-1 receptor stimulation that would worsen vasoconstriction, hypertension, and ischaemia.

🔑 KEY POINTS

1. The recognition of different toxidromes associated with common drug toxicity is essential to work out the underlying drug toxicity.
2. A 'drug screen' is not needed in most cases of poisoning
3. Beware of mixed poisoning and staggered overdose: always have a high index of suspicion.
4. In most cases the treatment of poisonings requires supportive therapy only, as specific antidotes are often not available. Liaise with the regional poisoning information centre as appropriate. Useful clinical information is available on the main TOXBASE web page: www.toxbase.org/ or mobile phone application.

CASE 80: GENERALISED RASH AND MALAISE

History

A 25-year-old man has presented to his general practitioner (GP) with a 1-month history of a generalised rash and pruritis. This rash started on the trunk and has spread to all four limbs, neck, and scalp. It is associated with malaise, recurrent fevers, and sweatiness. There are no mucosal ulcers or eye disorders. He does not recall any recent sore throat or flu-like illness. There is no drug or travel history, and he has no history of skin disorders. He works as a teacher and was fit and well prior to his present condition. However, he does have a 1-year history of back pain in the lumbar area and left knee pain, and as a result he has been unable to play football regularly.

Examination

This man feels extremely warm to the touch. There is a symmetrical, generalised body rash covering most of the body area with coarse scaling. There is no lymphadenopathy and no mouth ulcers, but his tongue is dry. His jugular venous pressure (JVP) is not seen even when lying flat, and his pulse is hyperdynamic but regular. The rest of the cardiovascular, respiratory, abdominal, and neurological examinations are unremarkable. Observations: temperature 37.7°C, heart rate 130 beats/min, blood pressure 110/70 mmHg, respiratory rate 24/min, SaO_2 100% on room air.

🔍 INVESTIGATIONS

		Normal range
White cells	15.0	$4-11 \times 10^9$/L
Haemoglobin	11.4	13–18 g/dL
Platelets	180	$150-400 \times 10^9$/L
Sodium	133	135–145 mmol/L
Potassium	3.4	3.5–5.0 mmol/L
Urea	12	3.0–7.0 mmol/L
Creatinine	140	60–110 µmol/L
C-reactive protein	88	<5 mg/L

? QUESTIONS

1. What is the most likely diagnosis?
2. What would be the appropriate management?

DOI: 10.1201/9781003241171-80

ANSWERS

This young man has presented with a rash, low-grade fever, and raised inflammatory markers. The generalised, scaly rash is typical for erythroderma. Other possible diagnoses could include a viral exanthem or a drug reaction (although there is no history of a new drug being introduced). Erythroderma is a clinical syndrome describing an erythematous rash involving more than 90% of the skin. This is a potentially life-threatening syndrome, as the extent of the rash can lead to skin failure: the skin is unable to maintain core temperature, retain fluid, and defend against infections.

A range of skin diseases can potentially lead to erythroderma, the most common being psoriasis, eczema and drug reactions, and rarely severe skin infections and T-cell lymphoma. Management includes general supportive care of skin failure (similar to that for a burn victim) as well as diagnosis and treatment of the underlying cause.

The diagnosis of the underlying cause of erythroderma should include a detailed history of the rash. A rapid onset with no preceding history may suggest an acute infection, allergy to environmental factors, or drugs. Usually erythrodermic patients have had a skin disease such as psoriasis or atopic eczema. A detailed drug and travel history should be recorded. Skin biopsies are often carried out when the diagnosis is unclear clinically. Cutaneous T-cell lymphoma is difficult to diagnose, and multiple skin biopsies are often done in order to firmly establish the diagnosis. The treatment of underlying severe psoriasis may involve an immunosuppressive agent such as methotrexate.

In this case the psoriasiform nature of the rash and history of preceding arthropathy point towards psoriasis as the underlying cause of his erythroderma.

General supportive care includes the following:

- Take steps to maintain the core temperature to prevent hypothermia.
- Stop all unnecessary medications.
- Give dietary supplements to support nutrition, as erythrodermic patients are in a high-catabolic state.
- Minimise the extent of intravenous access as much as possible.
- Give thromboprophylaxis unless clearly contraindicated.
- Assess fluid status by clinical examination and daily weighing to maintain good hydration, and manage renal failure accordingly.
- Monitor closely for clinical deterioration, as secondary sepsis is very common. Culture and manage with antibiotics.
- Prevent stress ulcers by proton pump inhibitors.
- Avoid blood glucose >10 mmol/L and manage with intravenous insulin accordingly.
- Give frequent attention to skin care. Apply emollients such as soft paraffin. Avoid adhesive tapes in affected skin areas. Frequently turn sedated/immobilised patients.
- Swab all affected areas frequently to look for bacterial superinfection and treat sepsis early and aggressively.
- Consider ophthalmic referral if the underlying cause has ophthalmic complications (e.g. toxic epidermal necrolysis).
- Pain and itching are often difficult to manage. Generous use of opioids and sedating antihistamines may be necessary.

🔑 **KEY POINTS**

1. Erythroderma is a clinical syndrome with a rash covering more than 90% of the body.
2. There is often a history of a previous skin disease, such as psoriasis or eczema.

CASE 81: COFFEE-GROUND VOMITING

History

A 78-year-old man has been admitted with a 1-day history of coffee-ground vomiting and black, tarry stools. His medical history is significant for hypertension and osteoarthritis. He regularly takes diclofenac 50 mg three times a day to control his knee pain, as well as aspirin 75 mg and bendroflumethiazide 2.5 mg once daily.

Examination

This man felt cool up to the wrists, and his pulse volume was reduced. His jugular venous pulse (JVP) was not visible. Respiratory and abdominal examinations were unremarkable. Per rectal examination confirmed fresh melaena. The patient's haemoglobin level on admission was 8.2 g/dL (normal range 13–17 g/dL).

Initial Treatment

An oesophagoduodenoscopy (OGD) was performed and showed a large duodenal ulcer with surrounding areas of bleeding. It was injected with adrenaline. He has been treated with intravenous proton pump inhibitors to aid ulcer healing. Twelve hours after his OGD he was found to have further melaena. He is feeling unwell and dizzy. Observations at this time: temperature 37.2°C, heart rate 128 beats/min irregular, blood pressure 100/65 mmHg, respiratory rate 24/min, SaO_2 98% on room air, Glasgow Coma Scale score 15/15.

🔍 INVESTIGATIONS

		Normal range
On admission (repeat samples awaited)		
White cells	7.2	4–11 × 10⁹/L
Haemoglobin	8.0	13–18 g/dL
Platelets	450	150–400 × 10⁹/L
Sodium	130	135–145 mmol/L
Potassium	3.2	3.5–5.0 mmol/L
Urea	24.0	3.0–7.0 mmol/L
Creatinine	180	60–110 µmol/L
C-reactive protein	10	<5 mg/L
Alanine aminotransferase	56	8–55 IU/L
Alkaline phosphatase	100	42–98 IU/L
INR	1.2	0.9–1.1
Arterial blood gas on room air:		
pH	7.35	7.35–7.45
pO₂	12.2	9.3–13.3 kPa
pCO₂	3.9	4.7–6.0 kPa
Lactate	3	<2 mmol/L
HCO₃	3	22–26 mmol/L
Base excess	−4	−3 to +3 mmol/L
Haemoglobin	6.2	13–18 g/dL

❓ QUESTION

1. What would be the appropriate management of this patient?

DOI: 10.1201/9781003241171-81

ANSWER

This man has had a further episode of melaena and, on examination, he is cool to the touch and shows signs of depleted fluid volume (reduced pulse volume and low JVP). The arterial blood gas sample shows an elevated lactate, an even lower haemoglobin, and a borderline metabolic acidosis, all of which are highly suggestive of rebleeding of the duodenal ulcer found on the OGD. The first management step is to resuscitate his hypovolaemic state and correct any clotting disorder that may contribute to his bleeding. The second step should include bleeding source control through repeat OGD.

The symptoms and signs are highly suggestive of hypovolaemia. It is important to support the circulation with intravenous fluid, so first ensure that multiple good intravenous accesses are available. The best intravenous fluid in this situation is red cell transfusion, so emergency cross-matching should be requested. Although the Hb is 8 g/dL and blood transfusion is recommended at the level of 7 g/dL, he is actively bleeding and hypovolaemic and is therefore likely to have a lower Hb once haemodynamic stability is achieved. In critical situations 'crash blood' can be used and is usually available in the accident and emergency department, labour ward, or the blood bank. In the interim, crystalloid fluid should be used to resuscitate the circulation. Bolus fluid challenge is preferable when blood pressure is unstable (e.g. 500 mL within 15 minutes). Where facilities allow, an arterial line should be inserted to allow continuous blood pressure monitoring. The target mean arterial pressure for resuscitation should not be excessively high to avoid exacerbating bleeding. Central venous access performed under ultrasound guidance should be considered in patients with another co-morbidity such as renal failure or congestive cardiac failure, although it is not the intravenous access of choice in urgent resuscitation, as it takes time to insert and the drip rate is lower than with a large-bore peripheral venous catheter. A urinary catheter should be inserted to monitor urine output and as a crude assessment of organ perfusion.

Since his pulse is irregular, a 12-lead ECG should be performed to look for arrhythmia such as atrial fibrillation. New atrial fibrillation in a critically unwell patient usually responds to treatment of the underlying cause—in this case hypovolaemia. Antiarrhythmic treatment should only be considered if the arrhythmia is impairing organ perfusion despite adequate fluid resuscitation. Amiodarone or digoxin should be used, as they have relatively mild or no negative inotropic effects.

In acute bleeding the target haemoglobin for transfusion is often set between 70 and 100 g/L, with a higher target range for those with a history of ischaemic heart disease. The clotting cascade should be optimised with products such as platelets, fresh frozen plasma, and cryoprecipitate to ensure platelets $>50 \times 10^9$/L, INR <1.4, and fibrinogen >1.4 g/L. Liaison with the haematology team is often helpful in these situations. Tranexamic acid is a potent fibrinolytic inhibitor which is cost-effective, but its efficacy has not been proven in the setting of upper gastrointestinal (UGI) bleeding. The use of tranexamic acid has increased since the publication of the CRASH-2 trial, which found a positive outcome with the use of tranexamic acid in trauma patients; however, the recently published HALT-IT trial suggested no benefit in severe cases of UGI bleed, so its use is currently not recommended routinely.

The optimal timing of proton pump inhibitor therapy initiation is currently not known with patients presenting with non-variceal bleeding. However, it is clear that, once a peptic ulcer is confirmed, a high-dose intravenous proton pump inhibitor (initial loading dose with continuous infusion for 72 hours) should be prescribed as soon as possible.

The Glasgow-Blatchford score is a validated system designed to predict the combined risk of requiring hospital-based intervention or mortality from UGI bleeding. As per the national guideline, it should be calculated at presentation of UGI bleed. If the Glasgow-Blatchford score ≤1 it might be clinically appropriate to consider outpatient UGI endoscopy. In patients deemed unwell enough to admit, it is ideally recommended that UGI endoscopy occur within 24 hours of presentation and even more urgently in ongoing bleed with haemodynamic instability.

While ongoing resuscitation takes place, the on-call endoscopist and surgeons should be contacted. Surgery may have a role in gastrointestinal bleeding when it is not controlled by endoscopy alone.

Helicobacter pylori is associated with 80%–95% of duodenal ulcers without a history of non-steroidal anti-inflammatory drug (NSAID) use. Its prevalence is lower in patients with duodenal ulcers related to NSAIDs. In the acute phase, empirical antibiotics are probably unnecessary, as they do not reduce the immediate bleeding risk. A CLO (*Campylobacter*-like organism) test is often carried out to detect *H. pylori* infection. Once tested positive, a triple therapy consisting of two antibiotics and an ulcer-healing agent should be started to reduce the future risk of ulcer reformation. Repeat OGD is often carried out with high-risk bleeding or rebleeding. However, in stable patients repeat OGD is necessary only with gastric ulcers to look for evidence of underlying malignancy.

 KEY POINTS

1. Rebleeding in the context of gastrointestinal bleeding carries significant mortality.
2. Prompt circulatory resuscitation and source control (endoscopy or surgery) should be carried out as soon as feasible.

CASE 82: BLURRED VISION WITH HEADACHE

History

A 32-year-old man attends the emergency department with a 2-day history of severe gener-alised headache. This is preceded by a 1-year history of intermittent throbbing headaches. There is no history of nausea, vomiting, epilepsy, muscle weakness, dizziness, hearing loss, or weight loss. He has no past medical history or drug history. He does not smoke or use recre-ational drugs. He drinks 8 units of alcohol per week.

Examination

The cardiorespiratory and abdominal examinations are unremarkable. There is no radio-femoral delay. He is alert and orientated, and there is no photophobia, neck stiffness, or rash. Cranial nerve and peripheral nervous system are within normal limits. Direct ophthalmos-copy shows bilateral papilloedema with multiple cotton-wool spots. Observations: temperature 36°C, heart rate 92 beats/min, blood pressure 260/140 mmHg, SpO_2 99% on room air.

INVESTIGATIONS

White cells	6.0
Haemoglobin	14.0
Platelets	200
Sodium	137
Potassium	3.7
Urea	12
Creatinine	162
Urine dipstick Protein	2+

? QUESTION

1. How would you manage this patient acutely?

ANSWER

This man presents with a hypertensive emergency, as evident by severe hypertension in the presence of target organ damage, which in this case is grade IV hypertensive retinopathy and acute kidney injury. Accelerated hypertension (malignant hypertension) is defined by severe hypertension with grade 3 or 4 retinopathy, nephropathy with or without microangiopathic haemolytic anaemia, or hypertensive encephalopathy.

The most important evaluation for severe hypertension (usually >180/120 mmHg) is to assess for the presence of target organ damage in the cardiovascular, renal, and central nervous system. Life-threatening target organ damage, which includes hypertensive encephalopathy, stroke, acute left ventricular failure, acute coronary syndrome, and aortic dissection, requires aggressive blood pressure lowering.

Assessment of target organ damage begins with history and examination for ischaemic heart disease, heart failure, peripheral vascular disease, cerebrovascular disease, polycystic kidneys, and hypertensive retinopathy. Perform a 12-lead ECG to look for voltage criteria of left ventricular hypertrophy, arrhythmias, previous myocardial infarction, or if the patient has chest pain, which is evidence of acute ischaemia. In this case, the urine sample should be sent for protein:creatinine ratio to formally evaluate for the severity of proteinuria. If there is haematuria, a sample should also be sent for microscopy. Blood film is required to determine the presence of microangiopathic haemolytic anaemia. A chest x-ray can demonstrate raised cardio-thoracic ratio and acute pulmonary oedema if the patient presents with symptoms of acute heart failure. All patients will require a transthoracic echocardiogram at a later stage to evaluate the left ventricular function and the presence of hypertrophy. Suspected cases of aortic dissection should be evaluated by CT aorta. Hypertensive encephalopathy occurs when the brain loses its ability to autoregulate its own perfusion in the context of severe hypertension. It leads to cerebral oedema and manifests as headache, nausea, vomiting, papilloedema, confusion, and seizure. Hypertensive encephalopathy is a diagnosis of exclusion, so neuroimaging (e.g. CT brain) should be requested to exclude stroke, encephalitis, or an intracranial space-occupying lesion. Symptoms of hypertensive encephalopathy rapidly resolve when blood pressure is lowered.

In all patients the lipid profile and glucose should be measured to look for other reversible cardiovascular risks. A pregnancy test should be carried out in women of childbearing age to exclude pre-eclampsia. Investigations for secondary causes of hypertension should be done in the context of accelerated hypertension and in a patient presenting with hypertension at a young age (<40 years). Of note, the prevalence of secondary hypertension is higher than previously thought, e.g. primary aldosteronism is found in 10% of all patients with hypertension, and up to 5% of hypertension cases is due to renal parenchymal/vascular disease. The secondary causes of hypertension investigations should at least include primary hyperaldosteronism (plasma renin and aldosterone), renovascular/parenchymal disease (renal ultrasound and other tests as guided by clinical findings), and phaeochromocytoma (plasma metanephrines or 24-hour urinary collection for metanephrines). Imaging for coarctation of the aorta and laboratory evaluation for other endocrine disease such as Cushing's syndrome can be considered on a case-by-case basis, depending on the initial clinical evaluation.

Intravenous antihypertensive treatment is only required when patients present with life-threatening end-organ damage. The initial aim of treatment is to lower blood pressure rapidly in a 2- to 6-hour timeframe under close supervision with invasive arterial blood pressure monitoring. The maximum initial fall in blood pressure at this point should not exceed 25% of the present value or below 160/100 mmHg. If the blood pressure falls too rapidly, it may cause organ ischaemia leading to stroke, myocardial infarction, or acute kidney injury. Patients with aortic dissection or haemorrhagic stroke have different targets, and local guidelines should be followed. In the absence of life-threatening end-organ damage, the elevated blood pressure does not need intravenous treatment, and it should be managed with oral antihypertensive therapy as per local guidelines. The aim is to lower blood pressure to 160/100 mmHg over the next 24–48 hours. This patient does not have life-threatening organ damage, but he has features of accelerated hypertension. He should be admitted for oral antihypertensive treatment with rapid dose titration. The presence of postural blood pressure drop is an indicator of hypovolaemia, which can develop after vasodilator treatment, and this requires correcting. Renal function should be closely monitored, and a reversible deterioration in renal function is expected when blood pressure is lowered. This usually corrects in the next few weeks. Renal function monitoring is also required when diuretics or angiotensin-converting enzyme inhibitors/angiotensin receptor blockers are prescribed.

 KEY POINTS

1. Severe hypertension is when blood pressure exceeds 180/120 mmHg. The type of intervention depends on the presence and severity of target organ damage.
2. Blood pressure lowering should be controlled to avoid precipitating organ ischaemia.

CASE 83: PRURITIC RASH AND ALOPECIA

History

A 73-year-old man attends the ambulatory clinic with a red, scaly rash over his body. For about 4 years he has had multiple, intensely itchy, red, scaly patches over his trunk. Despite skin biopsies on several occasions, the histological diagnosis of his condition remains inconclusive. A trial of a potent topical steroid in the past did not affect the patches. Over the past 2 weeks most areas of his body have become erythematous.

Examination

Cardiovascular and respiratory examinations are unremarkable. Abdominal examination reveals hepatosplenomegaly, and large lymph nodes are present in the axillary and cervical regions. Mucous membranes are normal. The entire surface area of the skin is diffusely erythematous. Palms and soles are thickened, and there is total alopecia. Observations: temperature 37.2°C, heart rate 110 beats/min, blood pressure 90/60 mmHg, SpO_2 96% on room air.

INVESTIGATIONS

White cells	15.0
Haemoglobin	9.4
Platelets	100
Sodium	133
Potassium	3.4
Urea	18
Creatinine	200
C-reactive protein	88

QUESTIONS

1. What is the unifying diagnosis?
2. What should be the immediate management?

DOI: 10.1201/9781003241171-83

ANSWERS

The history suggests that this man's rash has been going on for several years. The extent of the skin lesions is consistent with erythroderma, which is an acute dermatological emergency. Examination findings of hepatosplenomegaly and lymphadenopathy suggest a lymphoid organ infiltration. These features are highly suggestive of an underlying chronic cutaneous T-cell lymphoma: mycosis fungoides. The T cells involved are the circulating cutaneous lymphocyte-associated antigen positive (CLA+) cells, which home in on skin tissues and are usually CD4+ T cells. This is a rare disorder, and the erythroderma and infiltration of lymphoid organs are signs for the onset of Sézary's syndrome, the leukaemia variant of mycosis fungoides.

Definitive diagnosis can be difficult, and multiple biopsies may remain inconclusive for many years. Itchiness is a common complaint, and patients are often treated for other disorders such as eczema or psoriasis before a diagnosis can be made because of the wide variety of skin lesions patients can present with (e.g. plaques, scaly patches, and tumours). The staging of this disease depends on the tumour load in skin, blood, lymph node, and visceral organs: the management plan is dependent on the staging results. In this case, lymph node biopsy or bone marrow aspirate/biopsy may be helpful in confirming Sézary's syndrome. The general management of an acutely unwell erythrodermic patient is mentioned elsewhere in this book (see case 80). This patient should be referred to a dermatologist who will advise on the management of erythroderma and further investigations. General supportive care includes fluid resuscitation, nutritional support, monitoring of fluid and electrolyte balance, prevention of hypothermia, and vigilance on the signs and treatment of sepsis.

Owing to the wide variability in the presentation and natural history of this illness, treatment algorithms are not standardised. Possible treatment options are topical steroids, phototherapy, chemotherapy, radiotherapy, retinoids, photopheresis, immunobiological therapies, and bone marrow transplant in selected cases. Cutaneous T-cell lymphoma is an indolent illness that is not curable and can last for many years. However, patients with Sézary's syndrome have a poorer prognosis with a median survival of 1–3 years.

🔑 KEY POINTS

1. Mycosis fungoides is a cutaneous T-cell lymphoma, presenting with infiltration of lymphoid organs and skin changes.
2. The diagnosis can be difficult to make, and the disease can be very extensive by the time the diagnosis is reached.

CASE 84: ABDOMINAL PAIN, DIARRHOEA, AND FEVER

History

An 82-year-old man presented with a 3-day history of watery diarrhoea and fever. This was associated with worsening left-sided abdominal pain which started yesterday. It was described as constant and sharp and not relieved by defecation. This diarrhoea occurred up to ten times per day and was not associated with rectal bleeding. There was no recent travel history, and he had been cooking all his meals. His medical history includes hypertension, and he takes amlodipine 5 mg once daily.

Examination

This man showed no lymphadenopathy. Cardiorespiratory and neurological examinations were unremarkable. The abdomen was tender in the left iliac fossa with guarding and hyperactive bowel sounds. Observations: temperature 38.0°C, heart rate 100 beats/min, blood pressure 110/55 mmHg, respiratory rate 20/min, SaO_2 97% on room air.

Initial Treatment

The patient was admitted for intravenous antibiotics for presumptive diverticulitis. Twelve hours later he complains of worsening abdominal pain and new-onset left thigh pain. His abdomen is rigid with absent bowel sounds. His left iliac fossa and left thigh are very tender, with an extensive erythematous rash covering the left thigh from the knee up to the groin. New observations: temperature 39°C, heart rate 120 beats/min, blood pressure 98/55 mmHg, respiratory rate 24/min, SaO_2 97% on room air.

🔍 INVESTIGATIONS

		Normal range
White cells	32.0	$4\text{–}11 \times 10^9/L$
Haemoglobin	13.0	13–18 g/dL
Platelets	140	$150\text{–}400 \times 10^9/L$
Sodium	130	135–145 mmol/L
Potassium	2.8	3.5–5.0 mmol/L
Urea	12	3.0–7.0 mmol/L
Creatinine	120	60–110 µmol/L
C-reactive protein	458	<5 mg/L
INR	1.8	0.9–1.1
Arterial blood gas on room air:		
pH	7.37	7.35–7.45
pO_2	10.0	9.3–13.3 kPa
pCO_2	3.2	4.7–6.0 kPa
Lactate	6.0	<2 mmol/L
HCO_3	18	22–26 mmol/L
Base excess	−8	−3 to +3 mmol/L

DOI: 10.1201/9781003241171-84

? QUESTIONS

1. What is the most likely diagnosis?
2. How would you manage this condition?

ANSWERS

This man presented with diverticulitis, and one of the known complications is perforation. The finding of a new, tender, erythematous rash is worrying, as infected material from perforated bowel could potentially spread to surrounding soft tissues, leading to necrotising fasciitis.

The immediate management requires rapid stabilisation of septic shock using goal-directed therapy according to the Surviving Sepsis guidelines (www.sccm.org/SurvivingSepsisCampaign/Home). The rapidly progressing nature of necrotising fasciitis necessitates urgent surgical intervention for source control or debridement of necrotic tissue and resection of the affected bowel.

Necrotising fasciitis is a rapidly fatal condition affecting the skin. The offending organism(s) spread through the fascial compartments and release toxins. This leads to infective vasculitis and thrombus formation, resulting in vascular occlusion and tissue necrosis. This corresponds to a clinical finding of painful erythematous rash (sometimes bullous formation), which may progress to gangrenous discolouration if untreated. Crepitation is a classical finding but may not be present unless a gas-forming organism is involved.

Necrotising fasciitis can be divided into different types according to the microbiological agent(s) involved:

- Type 1 (polymicrobial)
- Type 2 (group A streptococcus)
- Type 3 (*Clostridia*—known to cause gas gangrene)
- Type 4 (fungal)

Mortality can approach 70%. Prompt surgical debridement is the key, and antibiotics alone are insufficient to alter the course of this illness.

In this case, the diagnosis of necrotising fasciitis was made, and the man went to theatre for debridement of the infected tissue. Despite the surgical intervention, the infection progressed and he developed a large deep vein thrombosis in his left leg. He ultimately required a left above-knee amputation. After intensive physiotherapy and assistance from the occupational therapists, he made a good recovery.

🔑 KEY POINTS

1. Necrotising fasciitis is a rapidly progressive and life-threatening condition affecting the skin and underlying tissues.
2. Surgical debridement plus antibiotic and fluid management will be necessary in order to remove any infected tissue.
3. Pain, swelling, and erythema over the area of infection are early signs and should raise the suspicion of necrotising fasciitis.

CASE 85: PROGRESSIVE DYSPHAGIA AND MUSCLE STIFFNESS

History

A 32-year-old man was admitted to a psychiatric ward 1 week earlier for inpatient treatment of acute psychosis. He was managed with haloperidol 5 mg intramuscularly every 8 hours and lorazepam 1 mg prn for sedation. He had been progressing well up until yesterday, when he complained of progressive dysphagia and muscle stiffness. Over the course of the day he developed a temperature (38.5°C) and has become increasingly drowsy.

Examination

This patient is drowsy. Cardiovascular, respiratory, and abdominal examinations are unremarkable. His Glasgow Coma Scale score is 11/15 (E3, V3, M5). Cranial nerve examination is difficult to perform, but no obvious abnormality is detected. The peripheral nervous system examination is significant for increased tone. Reflexes are difficult to elicit. He has had a low urine output. Observations: temperature 38.5°C, heart rate 120 beats/min, blood pressure 140/85 mmHg, SpO$_2$ 95% on room air

---

🔍 INVESTIGATIONS

White cells	16.0
Haemoglobin	15.0
Platelets	184
Sodium	135
Potassium	7.0
Urea	20
Creatinine	300
C-reactive protein	12
INR	1.1
Lactate dehydrogenase	1258
Creatine kinase	9988
Corrected Ca2+	1.9
Arterial blood gas on room air:	
pH	7.29
pO$_2$	14.0
pCO$_2$	3.5
Lactate	2.3
HCO$_3$	18
Base excess	−4
Urine dipstick	Blood 4+, protein 1+
ECG	Sinus tachycardia, with peaked T waves

❓ QUESTIONS

1. What is the most likely diagnosis?
2. How would you manage this patient?

DOI: 10.1201/9781003241171-85

ANSWERS

This man has findings consistent with neuroleptic malignant syndrome (NMS). NMS is rare, and only a small subset of patients is at risk. It usually presents within 3–9 days after initiation of antipsychotics or dose escalation, but patients remain at risk after chronic treatment. NMS is a medical emergency, and this patient's laboratory test shows acute kidney injury secondary to rhabdomyolysis, which is complicated by hyperkalaemia.

The diagnostic criteria for NMS are listed here in order of importance:

- Treatment with dopamine antagonist or abrupt withdrawal of dopamine agonist within 72 hours
- Temperature >38°C on two occasions
- Muscle rigidity
- Mental status alteration—confusion and/or decreased consciousness
- Creatinine kinase increased four times the upper limit of normal
- Autonomic instability with blood pressure fluctuation, sweating, and urinary incontinence
- Hypermetabolism (25% increase in heart rate and 50% increase in heart rate above baseline)
- Other causes, including toxic, metabolic, infectious, and neurological diseases, are excluded

Dopamine is central to thermoregulation and muscle tone. Blocking central dopaminergic receptors causes deranged temperature control and also direct toxicity to the muscle fibres, which leads to hyperthermia and muscle rigidity. The creatine kinase (CK) and lactate dehydrogenase (LDH) become elevated due to muscle cell necrosis. Rhabdomyolysis (the breaking down of muscle fibres) leads to the release of myoglobin, which precipitates an acute kidney injury. The finding of haematuria on urine dipstick is likely to be due to myoglobinuria rather than true haematuria. However, only 50% of patients present with myoglobinuria. The release of intracellular phosphate binds with calcium, leading to the observed hypocalcaemia. Treatment of hyperkalaemia should be urgent, but abnormal urate and calcium and phosphate levels are usually managed conservatively. It is also important to check the patient's INR, D-dimer level, fibrinogen level, and platelet count to look for evidence of disseminated intravascular coagulation (DIC), a known complication of severe rhabdomyolysis.

In this patient, the key priorities of his management should be (i) stopping the offending drugs and all other unnecessary medications that may worsen hyperkalaemia and renal function; (ii) aggressive fluid resuscitation with close fluid status monitoring; (iii) management of hyperkalaemia; and (iv) temperature control. He should be managed in a high-dependency area with airway monitoring, as he appeared drowsy on presentation. Full non-invasive cardiorespiratory monitoring is crucial to look for evidence of malignant arrhythmias secondary to hyperkalaemia. Intravenous access should be secured, and a bolus of crystalloid fluid challenge should be given in the first instance. Large-volume fluid replacement is likely to be required. Without delay, 10 mL of 10% calcium gluconate (or calcium chloride, whichever is accessible) should be given over 2–5 minutes, and 10 units of insulin with 20% glucose in 100 mL should be given over 5–15 minutes. Calcium gluconate should be repeated every 10 minutes until hyperkalaemic ECG changes are resolved. The effect of insulin/glucose should occur in 15 minutes and last for 4 hours. The maximum reduction of potassium is 1.0 mmol/L. Glucose should be monitored regularly, as hypoglycaemia could potentially be a problem up to 6 hours after insulin treatment. Urgent renal replacement therapy should be considered for refractory metabolic acidosis, hyperkalaemia, or anuria despite fluid resuscitation. Other treatment for NMS entails core temperature reduction using cooling devices, ice packs, fans, and cold intravenous fluids. Sedation with benzodiazepines is helpful in reducing muscle tone, distress, and temperature. Managing this patient's psychosis may be difficult, and close liaison with the psychiatry team may be necessary.

 KEY POINTS

1. NMS usually presents within 9 days of commencing antipsychotic medication.
2. Symptoms include pyrexia and rigidity, and management with fluids and cooling therapies should be commenced as soon as the diagnosis is made.

CASE 86: HEADACHE AND DOUBLE VISION

History

A 30-year-old woman had been experiencing a slowly progressive headache for the last few weeks. She described it as generalised. Over the last 24 hours she developed double vision prompting her presentation to A&E. On assessment in A&E, gross lower and upper limb neurology was intact but papilloedema was noted on fundoscopy. Past medical history only noted that she was on the combined oral contraceptive pill. She had no significant health conditions or family history. Observations revealed a HR 82 bpm, BP 110/64 mmHg, RR 12 breaths/min, oxygen saturations 98% on room air, temp 36.7°C, Glasgow Coma Scale (GCS) 15/15. In view of the papilloedema, she underwent a contrast-enhanced CT head scan that was unremarkable for a space-occupying lesion or intracranial bleed but showed a suggestion of filling defect in the sagittal vein.

? | **QUESTIONS**

1. How would you manage this patient?
2. What other conditions should be considered?

ANSWERS

1. The patient had symptoms and signs of raised intracranial pressure, but a bleed or space-occupying lesion were ruled out on the CT head scan. A subsequent MRI brain with venogram confirmed sagittal vein thrombosis. Although headache is the most common symptom, neurological features may complicate the presentation, including stroke (ischaemic or haemorrhagic) and seizures, depending on the extent of thrombosis and its location in the veins and sinuses. In this case, anticoagulation is required with either low-molecular-weight heparin or unfractionated heparin. Further management should include blood tests to look for prothrombotic conditions and thrombophilias. Any medications that increase thrombotic risk should be enquired about and stopped if possible. She is on an oestrogen-containing contraceptive pill. Other risk factors include pregnancy and malignancy. In some cases it might be possible to perform endovascular thrombolysis or thrombectomy if systemic anticoagulation is contraindicated or in severe cases. Long-term anticoagulation with vitamin K antagonists is required. The exact duration depends on cause.

   Cerebral venous thrombosis (CVT) is rare but a recognised cause of stroke (0.5% of all cases). It tends to occur in a younger age group, being more common in females. Most cases have a good prognosis, but around 10%–15% have a severe complication, including stroke or death.

2. CVT can present with headaches or other neurological signs that can mimic migraine, other causes of raised intracranial pressure, stroke, meningism, and encephalopathy. Often imaging with CT/MRI brain with blood tests and lumber puncture as required can rule out other causes.

 KEY POINTS

1. Sagittal venous thrombosis is a rare but recognised cause of stroke.
2. MRI with MR brain venogram is the most sensitive investigation to identify cerebral venous sinus thrombosis.

CASE 87: DEFECTIVE VISION AND EYE PAIN

History

A 24-year-old woman has presented to the emergency department with a reduction in visual acuity of her right eye, developing over the past few days. This is associated with pain on right eye movement, and she describes a reduction in colour vision in the same eye. She denies any headache or other neurological symptoms.

Examination

This young woman's right and left eye visual acuities are 6/24 and 6/6, respectively. Examination of the visual fields reveals a central scotoma. There is a relative afferent pupillary defect on the right eye. Fundoscopy reveals a normal optic disc. The rest of the cardiorespiratory, abdominal, and neurological examinations are unremarkable.

? QUESTIONS

1. What is the diagnosis?
2. How can this condition be managed?

ANSWERS

Presentation of reduced visual acuity and colour vision is typical of any optic neuropathy (except for papilloedema: usually patients suffering from papilloedema do not complain of reduced visual acuity). In common with all optic neuropathies, there is a varying degree of relative afferent pupillary defect and central scotoma. It is also important to perform a fundoscopy to exclude retinal pathologies (e.g. retinal detachment), which can present in a similar way. In this scenario the patient is likely to have experienced an episode of optic neuritis or retrobulbar neuritis.

When patients over the age of 50 years present with symptoms of optic neuropathy, it is essential to ask whether there has been any history of headache or polymyalgia symptoms (e.g. shoulder and/or pelvic girdle pain) and to measure the erythrocyte sedimentation rate (ESR) to exclude temporal arteritis. Although rare, severe sphenoidal sinusitis can also present with a sudden reduction in visual acuity and colour vision and pain on eye movement. If this is suspected, an urgent CT of the sinus cavities and an ear/nose/throat (ENT) opinion should be sought.

Optic neuritis typically affects young females and rarely presents over the age of 45 years. The classical presenting symptoms are of unilateral loss of visual acuity and pain on eye movement. It is usually self-limiting, with full function returning within 3 months. The cause is often not identified and labelled as idiopathic in the absence of other evidence of a systemic process. However, 50% of patients will develop a second episode of optic neuritis, and this is highly suggestive of multiple sclerosis, which should be further investigated. It is therefore important that the presence of paraesthesia, dizziness, shooting neck pain or limb weakness, and Uthoff's phenomenon (worsening of neurological symptoms in warm conditions, e.g. a hot bath) guides you towards the diagnosis of multiple sclerosis in patients who present with optic neuritis.

The treatment of acute optic neuritis can include steroids; however, it is best to refer to local policy and follow specialist advice.

🔑 **KEY POINTS**

1. Optic neuritis presents with pain, loss of vision, and a reduction in colour vision (particularly the colour red).
2. Optic neuritis is often a feature of multiple sclerosis, so a full history must be taken and a neurological examination should be performed.

History

A 52-year-old man has presented to his general practitioner (GP) with a 4-month history of back pain. This is associated with recurrent fever and weight loss of 4 kg over the previous 4 months. The back pain has been gradually getting worse and is now constant, radiating to the front of his chest. It is made worse on lifting and movement and is only mildly alleviated by paracetamol and ibuprofen. He is normally fit and well. He cannot recall any trauma or heavy lifting that might have triggered this pain. He was born in India and has not left the UK since becoming a resident in 1976.

Examination

There is no lymphadenopathy. Cardiorespiratory, abdominal, and neurological examinations are unremarkable. There is general tenderness around the thoracic spine extending down to the upper lumbar region. There is no neurological deficit. Rectal examination is normal. A chest x-ray reveals a calcified nodule in the upper zone. A spinal x-ray is shown in Figure 88.1. Observations: temperature 37.5°C, heart rate 96 beats/min, blood pressure 120/80 mmHg, SaO$_2$ 99% on room air.

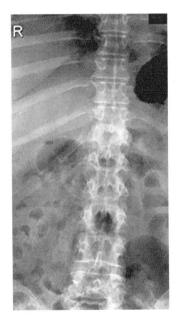

Figure 88.1

DOI: 10.1201/9781003241171-88

INVESTIGATIONS

		Normal range
White cells	14.0	$4-11 \times 10^9$/L
Haemoglobin	12.8	13–18 g/dL
Platelets	400	$150-400 \times 10^9$/L
Sodium	140	135–145 mmol/L
Potassium	3.9	3.5–5.0 mmol/L
Urea	4.0	3.0–7.0 mmol/L
Creatinine	76	60–110 µmol/L
Corrected calcium	2.3	2.2–2.6 mmol/L
C-reactive protein	38	<5 mg/L
Erythrocyte sedimentation rate	45	Male, age/2; female, [age+10]/2 mm/h

QUESTION

1. What are the possible causes of this man's symptoms and investigation findings?

ANSWER

This man has presented with back pain associated with 'red flag' symptoms. When evaluating back pain, the red flags that are important to explore are:

- First back pain at age <20 or >55
- Non-mechanical back pain (stiffness at rest)
- Thoracic back pain
- Past history of cancer
- History or examination findings suggesting immunosuppression (e.g. oropharyngeal candidiasis, oral hairy leucoplakia, Kaposi's sarcoma)
- Systemic symptoms (e.g. weight loss, night sweats, fever, rigor)
- Abnormal neurology (e.g. abnormal bowel and bladder functions, abnormal sensation and coordination, muscular weakness)
- Structural spinal defect and severe localised tenderness, especially in the thoracic region

For these scenarios, further investigations should be targeted to look for possible underlying infections or malignancy.

This patient's chest radiograph shows a calcified nodule in the upper lobe, indicating old primary tuberculosis. The spine radiograph in Figure 88.1 shows partial collapse of T11 and T12 with loss of the intervening disc space. These findings and systemic symptoms raise the possibility of Pott's disease (spinal tuberculosis), although other infection or malignancies cannot be completely excluded. The possible findings of vertebral osteomyelitis on plain radiography are bony destruction, wedge fractures, and lytic or sclerotic lesions. If spinal cord compression is suspected, an urgent MRI of the spine and urgent referral to spinal surgeons should be organised. Any delay could potentially increase the possibility of permanent disability. Infections in the spine tend to involve the intervertebral discs early, whereas malignancy tends to affect the vertebrae themselves, often sparing the discs.

Over 50% of vertebral osteomyelitis is caused by *Staphylococcus aureus* and tuberculosis. Pott's disease is most common over the thoracic region and can extend over several segments and through intravertebral foramina into the pleura, peritoneum, or psoas muscles. If tuberculosis is suspected, then HIV testing should be considered, as tuberculosis is more common in immunocompromised people. MRI of the spine is particularly helpful to look for osteomyelitis, a paraspinal tumour or abscess, and spinal cord compression. Histology or microbiology samples should be taken to confirm the diagnosis whenever possible. Treatment should be directed towards the underlying aetiology. Prolonged antibiotics will be required. Surgical intervention, including debridement and/or correction of complications, may also be necessary.

> 🔑 **KEY POINTS**
>
> 1. It is important to enquire about the 'red flag' symptoms when evaluating back pain to ensure serious disorders are not missed.
> 2. A prolonged course of antibiotics is required with a combined management approach of both medical and surgical intervention if necessary.

CASE 89: ABDOMINAL PAIN FOLLOWING ALCOHOL BINGE

History

A 48-year-old man has presented with recurrent vomiting after a large binge of alcohol intake 24 hours ago. Over the last hour he has become short of breath with a new dry cough. This is associated with severe epigastric pain, which is constant and radiating towards his right chest. He is normally fit and well and has no past medical history.

Examination

This man looks unwell and is cool to the touch. His jugular venous pulse (JVP) is not seen. There is no lymphadenopathy. His pulse volume is reduced, and his capillary refilling time is 4 seconds. There is crepitus felt on palpation of the skin around the right neck extending to the chest wall. His chest is dull to percussion on the right. Auscultation of the chest reveals air entry bilaterally with reduced breath sounds and a pleural rub on the right side. His upper abdomen is very tender with absent bowel sounds. An ECG reveals sinus tachycardia. Observations: temperature 37.8°C, heart rate 130 beats/min, blood pressure 90/60 mmHg, respiratory rate 28/min, SaO2 92% on room air.

🔍 INVESTIGATIONS

Arterial blood gas on room air:		Normal range
pH	7.28	7.35–7.45
pO_2	7.9	9.3–13.3 kPa
pCO_2	3.1	4.7–6.0 kPa
Lactate	8.0	<2 mmol/L
HCO_3	16	22–26 mmol/L
Base excess	−9	−3 to +3 mmol/L

❓ QUESTIONS

1. What are the differential diagnoses?
2. How would you resuscitate this man?

ANSWERS

This man is moribund, and appropriate resuscitation should be instigated immediately. His breathing should be supported with oxygen, and his circulation should be fluid resuscitated.

The differential diagnoses are cardiogenic, hypovolaemic, or septic shock. The clinical presentation and the ECG findings are not consistent with cardiogenic shock. The history of recurrent vomiting, lower chest pain, and subcutaneous emphysema—the Mackler triad—is consistent with Boerhaave's syndrome (spontaneous oesophageal perforation). Gastric contents spill over into the mediastinum to cause acute mediastinitis and erosions of the surrounding structures and pleural effusion or hydropneumothorax. It is important to keep the patient 'nil by mouth'. An urgent plain film or CT with water-soluble contrast often confirms the diagnosis. The timing of imaging is sometimes difficult in critically unwell patients, and patients should be adequately resuscitated to minimise the chance of deterioration in transit and at the radiology department. In this case a gastrografin swallow confirms an oesophageal leak into the right chest cavity (see Figure 89.1).

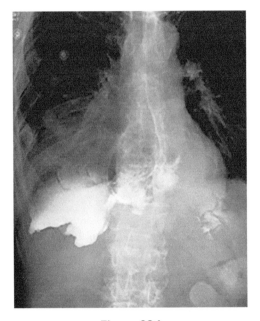

Figure 89.1

Other potential causes of oesophageal perforation are foreign-body ingestion and oesophageal instrumentation (e.g. oesophagogastroduodenoscopy, especially in pre-existing oesophageal lesions such as cancers). Usually the patient is gravely ill. The abdomen may be rigid, leading to a false diagnosis of perforated duodenal ulcer. The pathophysiology of Boerhaave's syndrome is not fully understood, but the lack of serosa in the oesophagus increases the likelihood of rupture. Broad-spectrum antibiotics should be given immediately, and urgent surgical review should be sought. The mortality of this condition is up to 40% if it is not managed promptly and appropriately.

🔑 KEY POINTS

1. The definitive treatment for a perforated viscus is surgical intervention.
2. It is important, however, to optimise the patient's condition prior to surgery through appropriate fluid resuscitation and antibiotic therapy.

CASE 90: ABDOMINAL PAIN, MALAISE, AND FEVER

History

A 41-year-old woman has presented to the emergency department with an acute-onset right flank pain radiating to her right iliac fossa that woke her from her sleep 4 hours ago. The pain is increasingly severe, and she is finding it hard to stay still. The pain is associated with nausea and vomiting. In the last few minutes she begins to have chills and rigour. There is no recent change in bowel habit. She was admitted 3 months ago with pyelonephritis, but she is otherwise fit and well and does not take any regular medications. Her last menstrual period was 17 days ago.

Examination

This woman is not icteric, and there is no lymphadenopathy. Her cardiorespiratory examination is unremarkable. On palpation of her abdomen, there is tenderness, which is worse in the right flank. There is no rebound tenderness. Bowel sounds are normal. Rectal examination reveals an empty rectum. Observations: temperature 39°C, heart rate 110 beats/min, blood pressure 100/60 mmHg, respiratory rate 24/min, SpO$_2$ 100% on room air.

🔍 INVESTIGATIONS

White cells	18.0
Haemoglobin	15.6
Platelets	208
Sodium	134
Potassium	3.5
Urea	4.0
Creatinine	112
Bilirubin	10
Alanine aminotransferase	16
Alkaline phosphatase	70
Albumin	38
C-reactive protein	120
Amylase	88
Urine dipstick:	
—Protein	2+
—Blood	4+
—Nitrite	Positive
—Leu	4+
Urinary pregnancy test	Negative

❓ QUESTIONS

1. What is the diagnosis?
2. How would you manage this woman?

DOI: 10.1201/9781003241171-90

ANSWERS

This woman has acute renal colic complicated by sepsis secondary to an obstructing stone. The presence of right flank pain radiating to the right iliac fossa may point to mid-ureteral renal stones. Other diagnoses that can cause a similar presentation are biliary sepsis, appendicitis, and ectopic pregnancy, but they are very unlikely here given the normal liver function test, negative pregnancy test, and evidence of renal stones/urinary tract infection on urine dipstick. A pregnancy test should be carried out in all women of childbearing potential presenting with abdominal and flank pain.

CT kidney, ureter, and bladder (CT-KUB) is considered the gold-standard investigation for renal stones. It can also examine other abdominal organs for alternative diagnoses. Ultrasound is an alternative especially in pregnant women, but it is less sensitive than CT-KUB for renal stones. Ultrasound KUB can detect pyelonephritis, abscess, and the presence of hydronephrosis. Other investigations should include serum calcium, phosphate, urate, urine, and blood cultures.

Renal colic is a very painful condition, and opioid analgesia in additional to paracetamol will be required. Non-steroidal anti-inflammatory drugs are also effective, but care must be taken in the context of obstructive nephropathy. Fluid resuscitation and empirical antibiotics for pyelonephritis should be given according to local policy. Urinary output should be monitored. Urgent urology consultation is required to consider surgical decompression to relieve the ureteric obstruction.

Calcium stones contribute to 80% of renal stones. The other common stones are urate (10%), cystine (1%), and struvite (up to 5%). Cystine stones reflect an underlying inborn error of metabolism, and patients may have a positive family history. Struvite stones are infection stones. Advice for secondary prevention or renal stones include drinking 2.5–3L of water each day and reducing salt intake to 6 g/day, as sodium causes hypercalciuria. Patients with urate stones should consume a low-purine diet.

🔑 **KEY POINTS**

1. Renal stones accompanied by sepsis is a urological emergency.
2. In female patients of childbearing age, a pregnancy test should be performed to ensure an ectopic pregnancy is not missed.

CASE 91: RESPIRATORY DISTRESS AND OEDEMA

History

A 78-year-old woman has presented to the emergency department with acute severe shortness of breath and wheeze, which is increasingly severe. She has no chest pain, cough, or fever. Her medical history includes hypertension, peripheral vascular disease, and chronic kidney disease stage 4. Over the past year her estimated glomerular filtration rate has deteriorated by two-thirds, and her hypertension has become more treatment-resistant, accompanied by reduced exercise tolerance, orthopnoea, and bilateral lower limb oedema. Of note, this is her third similar presentation to the hospital in the past year. She is taking several drugs: hydralazine 25 mg thrice daily; isosorbide mononitrate 60 mg once daily; nebivolol 5 mg once daily; spironolactone 25 mg once daily; furosemide 80 mg twice daily; amlodipine 10 mg once daily; aspirin 75 mg once daily; atorvastatin 10 mg once daily. She has no known drug allergies.

Examination

This elderly woman is in respiratory distress, and immediate high-flow oxygen is provided. There is peripheral oedema up to her knees. Her pulse is regular, with jugular venous pressure (JVP) raised at 11 cm. On auscultation her heart sounds are normal. There are inspiratory crackles up to the mid-zone bilaterally and mild end-expiratory wheeze. Echocardiography 1 month prior to the current presentation showed moderate concentric left ventricular hypertrophy, normal left ventricular size and function, and grade 2 diastolic dysfunction. A chest x-ray is shown in Figure 91.1. Observations: temperature 37°C, heart rate 106 beats/min, blood pressure 160/100 mmHg, respiratory rate 38/min, SpO_2 90% on room air.

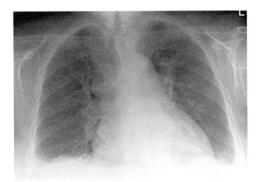

Figure 91.1

DOI: 10.1201/9781003241171-91

INVESTIGATIONS

Haemoglobin	12
White cell count	6.1
Platelets	165
Sodium	135
Potassium	5.0
Urea	7.2
Creatinine	162
C-reactive protein	<5

Urine dipstick:
Protein 1+ Blood   Nitrite negative, leucocyte negative
12-lead ECG   Sinus tachycardia. Voltage criteria for
                          left ventricular hypertrophy. No acute
                          ischaemic changes.

QUESTIONS

1. What is the differential diagnosis?
2. What is the appropriate management?

ANSWERS

The differential diagnoses of acute shortness of breath and wheeze include acute exacerbation of obstructive airway diseases and acute pulmonary oedema. In this case the history, examination, and chest x-ray findings are consistent with acute pulmonary oedema. Note the upper-lobe blood diversion and the alveolar infiltrates throughout the lung fields suggestive of pulmonary oedema, as well as the blunted costophrenic angles, indicating small pleural effusions, which are all due to fluid overload.

The immediate treatments for acute pulmonary oedema include high-flow oxygen and ventilatory support, diuretics, and vasodilators. Routine use of morphine/diamorphine is not recommended due to adverse outcomes in observational studies. In this case high-flow oxygen should be administered and non-invasive continuous positive airway pressure (CPAP) ventilation should be considered, as this patient is in respiratory distress (respirate rate >25 beats/min and SpO_2 <90%). Intravenous furosemide and glyceryl trinitrate are the mainstay treatments to relieve fluid retention and reduce the left ventricular preload and afterload. Venous thromboembolism prevention is important in this group of patients.

It is always important to look for the underlying causes of acute pulmonary oedema such as acute coronary syndrome or arrhythmia. Her echocardiogram 1 month before this presentation showed a preserved left ventricular ejection fraction despite two previous presentations of acute heart failure. In fact, this patient meets the diagnostic criteria for heart failure with preserved ejection fraction (HFpEF), which are (i) symptoms and signs of heart failure, (ii) left ventricular ejection fraction >50%, and (iii) objective evidence of structural and functional abnormalities consistent with the presence of left ventricular diastolic dysfunction and raised left ventricular filling pressures. HFpEF is common and present in 50% of heart failure patients. In this case, the underlying aetiology is resistant hypertension. There is no specific treatment for HFpEF other than to optimise lifestyle measures (e.g. smoking cessation, weight loss), treat hypertension, monitor fluid status, treat diabetes mellitus (if present), and follow the lipid profile. The sodium glucose co-transport 2 inhibitors may have a role in the treatment of HFpEF.

This patient's recent history of resistant hypertension, worsening renal impairment, fluid retention, proteinuria, and recurrent presentations of pulmonary oedema are collectively pointing towards renovascular disease as the underlying aetiology of her recent deterioration. 'Flash pulmonary oedema' is a term used to describe circulatory overload out of proportion to left ventricular systolic function and is often ascribed to underlying haemodynamically significant bilateral renal artery stenosis (RAS).

RAS is sometimes found incidentally on angiography performed for another reason, and not all lesions (especially those with <50% lumen occlusion) cause secondary hypertension or renal disease. About 90% of RAS is caused by atherosclerosis, and the remainder is due to fibromuscular dysplasia (FMD). This patient is most likely to have atherosclerotic RAS, as FMD usually presents as secondary hypertension at a young age and is not usually accompanied by renal impairment or heart failure. The treatment for FMD is percutaneous renal angioplasty, and patients usually respond well to this. Screening for FMD in carotid or vertebral arteries is recommended if renal FMD is found. By contrast, the treatment of atherosclerotic RAS remains a topic of debate, as not all patients achieve better control of blood pressure or recovery of renal function following intervention. Renal angioplasty in this group carries significant risks, including irreversible cholesterol embolisation and renal artery thrombosis or rupture. Therefore, renal angioplasty should only be considered on a case-by-case basis in patients with (i) recurrent acute heart failure, (ii) declining renal function in the context of bilateral RAS or

RAS affecting solitary function kidney, and (iii) refractory hypertension. The main treatments for atherosclerotic RAS are similar to atherosclerotic disease in other arterial territories, which include lifestyle modifications (smoking cessation, salt intake <6 g/day, and weight loss) and control of blood pressure, glucose, and cholesterol. A combination of antihypertensives is often needed to adequately control blood pressure in atherosclerotic RAS. Angiotensin-converting enzyme (ACE) inhibitors or angiotensin receptor blockers (ARBs) should be used with caution, with interval renal profile monitoring (e.g. 1 week after initiation and change in dose). Dose should be withheld in significant hyperkalaemia and/or in the presence of >30% increase in serum creatinine or >25% fall in estimated glomerular filtration rate from baseline.

🔑 KEY POINTS

1. Acute pulmonary oedema is a common medical emergency that should be promptly recognised and treated.
2. The definitive treatment of atherosclerotic RAS remains controversial. Control of reversible cardiovascular risk such as smoking cessation, cholesterol, and blood pressure lowering may slow down the progression of renovascular disease.

CASE 92: NIGHT SWEATS, POLYURIA, AND POLYDIPSIA

History

A 75-year-old man has presented to the ambulatory clinic with a 1-month history of dry cough, reduced exercise tolerance due to exertional shortness of breath, and unintentional weight loss. These symptoms are associated with night sweats, polyuria, and polydipsia. For the past week his urine has become very dark and discoloured. His history includes hypertension, which was well controlled until 4 months ago. He does not smoke or drink alcohol. His drug history includes chlortalidone 25 mg once daily.

Examination

This man is not icteric. There is no lymphadenopathy. Coarse inspiratory crackles are heard on auscultation of the lower zones bilaterally. Abdominal examination reveals a large right-sided varicocoele that does not collapse when lying supine. The rest of the examination is unremarkable. A chest x-ray is shown in Figure 92.1. Observations: temperature 37.6°C, heart rate 104 beats/min, blood pressure 190/110 mmHg, SpO$_2$ 94% on room air.

🔍 INVESTIGATIONS

White cells	12.2
Haemoglobin	10.8
Platelets	333
Sodium	136
Potassium	3.4
Urea	10
Creatinine	120
C-reactive protein	72
INR	1.0
Corrected calcium	3.0
Urine	Blood 4+, protein 1+

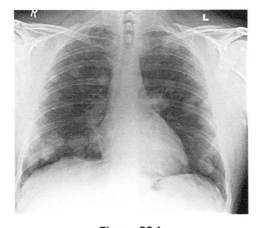

Figure 92.1

? QUESTIONS

1. What are the differential diagnoses?
2. What further investigations should be performed?

ANSWERS

The chest radiograph shows multiple, well-defined, rounded opacities that may explain his symptoms of shortness of breath and dry cough. Malignancies should be considered for multiple 'coin'-shaped opacities on a chest radiograph, especially when there are also complaints of night sweats and weight loss. Renal cell carcinomas (RCCs) are one of the most common sources of large pulmonary (cannonball) metastases. Sometimes it may be difficult to decide whether there is bacterial pneumonia that has superinfected the underlying malignancy, especially when there are pneumonic symptoms (fever, productive cough, and shortness of breath) and raised inflammatory markers (which can be raised solely due to malignancy). If there is enough suspicion for superinfection, empirical antibiotics should be started.

The dark urine is likely macroscopic haematuria, and this is a symptom of urological malignancy until proven otherwise, although rarely glomerulonephritis can present in this way. The classical presentation triad for RCC is macroscopic haematuria, flank pain, and palpable mass. In reality patients rarely present with all three symptoms and signs: approximately 50% of patients are asymptomatic. Patients with RCC may also present with persistent microscopic haematuria, so this is a reason for investigation for possible underlying urological malignancy. RCC may secret several hormones, including parathyroid hormone– related peptide, adrenocorticotrophic hormone, erythropoietin and vasopressin leading to hypercalcaemia, Cushing's syndrome, polycythaemia, and syndrome of inappropriate antidiuretic hormone. Other paraneoplastic conditions are Stauffer's syndrome (liver failure without liver metastasis) and myoneuropathies. Varicocoeles are a common condition that affects 10% of males. Ninety per cent of varicocoeles occur on the left, and this may be due to the difference in venous drainage of the two sides. The left testicular vein drains into the high-pressure renal vein, whereas the right testicular vein drains directly into the inferior vena cava. When these drainages are obstructed by tumours such as RCC, it may present as varicocoele. Such varicocoeles may not collapse when lying supine—a pointer towards further investigation for underlying invasive malignancy. A short history of varicocoele, especially on the right side, should also trigger further investigation for underlying malignancy.

The history of polyuria and polydipsia is consistent with the finding of moderate hypercalcaemia. This should be treated with intravenous fluid replacement in the first 24 hours with close fluid status monitoring for fluid overload, especially in older people. Bisphosphonates should be given if intravenous fluid is insufficient. This will take at least 48 hours to achieve a significant reduction in plasma calcium level.

The main investigation for RCC is CT scan of chest, abdomen, and pelvis for staging and to evaluate local anatomy. A bone scan should be considered if bone metastasis is likely. Biopsy can be obtained from the most accessible metastatic lesions in advanced disease. Radical nephrectomy with curative intent is achievable in localised RCC only. In advanced disease, treatment options include vascular endothelial growth factor inhibitors and immune checkpoint inhibitors.

 KEY POINT

1. Hypercalcaemia is a common oncological emergency that should be screened for and treated appropriately.

CASE 93: PAINFUL SHOULDER AND MALAISE

History

A 62-year-old woman with a background history of rheumatoid arthritis attends the emergency department with a 1-week history of painful right shoulder. This has gradually worsened, and she is unable to move her shoulder owing to severe pain. This is associated with worsening general malaise. Her medical history includes stage 3 chronic kidney disease. She takes methotrexate 10 mg once a week, folic acid 5 mg once a week, and ramipril 5 mg daily.

Examination

This woman is obese, but cardiorespiratory and abdominal examinations are unremarkable. Her right shoulder joint is tender on palpation, and no active or passive movements are possible because of pain. There is mild erythema over the right shoulder, and it feels slightly warm to the touch. A shoulder x-ray reveals osteopenic bones, but no joint abnormality is detected. Observations: temperature 37.9°C, heart rate 92 beats/min, blood pressure 100/65 mmHg, SpO$_2$ 93% on room air.

INVESTIGATIONS

White cells	8.0
Haemoglobin	9.0
Platelets	155
Sodium	135
Potassium	3.7
Urea	9
Creatinine	142
C-reactive protein	46

QUESTIONS

1. What are the main differential diagnoses in this case?
2. What would be your immediate management plan?

DOI: 10.1201/9781003241171-93

ANSWERS

The main differential diagnoses of this woman's presentation are septic arthritis, pathological fracture, crystal arthropathies, or acute flare of rheumatoid arthritis. Septic arthritis should be suspected in any patient with rheumatoid arthritis with sudden onset or worsening of joint symptoms. Clinical signs of septic arthritis may be atypical or may not reflect the severity due to concomitant immunosuppressive therapy—in this case with methotrexate. There is an increased risk of pathological or low-impact fractures in rheumatoid arthritis owing to the underlying inflammatory process, inactivity, and long-term exposure to systemic corticosteroids.

It is prudent to rule out septic arthritis in the first instance. Obtain blood tests to look for raised inflammatory markers and to look for other target damage such as chronic kidney disease, which may be relevant in a multi-system disorder associated with frequent use of immunosuppressives.

Interpretation of C-reactive protein (CRP) and erythrocyte sedimentation rate (ESR) may be difficult, particularly the ESR. Chronic anaemia is common in patients with rheumatoid arthritis, and ESR is raised in anaemia. Both CRP and ESR could be raised due to underlying inflammation, or they could be mildly raised due to immunosuppressive therapy.

Blood culture should be obtained if pyrexial. Joint aspiration should be carried out as soon as possible but should not delay the administration of empirical antibiotics. Joint aspirate should be sent for microscopy for bacteria and culture and for crystal identification. The joint should be aspirate to dryness to remove infection and to relieve joint pain. If a prosthetic joint is involved, then aspiration should be carried out in an operating theatre by an orthopaedic surgeon.

Once the diagnosis of septic arthritis is confirmed, a joint washout should be considered. In this scenario methotrexate should be withdrawn temporarily. Pain management is important, so paracetamol and opioids should be considered as appropriate. Staphylococci or streptococci are the most common bacteria causing septic arthritis, accounting for >90% of the cases. Empirical intravenous antibiotics should cover these organisms, and a prolonged course of antibiotics is required in most cases.

🔑 KEY POINTS

1. Patients with known rheumatoid arthritis presenting with acute joint pain should be investigated for septic arthritis.
2. If the diagnosis of septic arthritis is confirmed, a joint washout should be considered. If this is not appropriate, repeat joint aspirate to dryness may be required.
3. Pain management is important, so paracetamol and opioids should be considered as appropriate.

CASE 94: FACIAL RASH

History

A 34-year-old woman has presented to her general practitioner (GP) with a 1-day history of high fever, lethargy, and a rapidly spreading rash over the malar bones and nasal bridges. She has a 5-year history of systemic lupus erythematosus (SLE) that had initially presented with inflammation and pain of the small joints of the hands, but this is now well-controlled by hydroxychloroquine. She has been monitored by a rheumatologist over the past 5 years, and, apart from a mild anaemia, she has had no other systemic features of SLE. She does not have a history of recent foreign travel.

Examination

This woman is warm to the touch, her pulse is bounding, and she looks unwell. Over the nasal bridge and malar bones there is a well-demarcated erythematous plaque that is tender. There are no oral lesions, but there are multiple small cervical lymph nodes. The rest of the examination is unremarkable. Observations: temperature 38.7°C, heart rate 110 beats/min, blood pressure 100/60 mmHg, respiratory rate 24/min, SpO_2 96% on room air.

INVESTIGATIONS

White cells	15.0
Haemoglobin	10.0
Platelets	100
Sodium	137
Potassium	4.1
Urea	10
Creatinine	140
C-reactive protein	120
Erythrocyte sedimentation rate	100 mm/h

? QUESTION

1. How would you manage this woman?

DOI: 10.1201/9781003241171-94

ANSWER

SLE is a complex multi-system disorder that carries excess mortality. The majority of SLE patients have a natural history of episodic exacerbations or flares. Sometimes remissions may be prolonged, and the pattern of exacerbations is usually established within 5–10 years of disease onset. If aggressive SLE flares occur frequently and early in the disease course, then mortality risk is high. Premature cardiovascular disease (stroke, ischaemic heart disease), thromboembolism, osteoporosis, lupus nephritis, susceptibility to infection, and elevated risks for haematological malignancies and solid tumours (lung, thyroid, and vulval) are major complications associated with SLE, accounting for the 2.6-fold increase in all-cause mortality compared to the general population.

When reviewing a patient with a history of SLE, the main focus is to decide whether the presentation is due to a flare or to a complication of SLE such as infection or an unrelated condition. In this scenario it is important to decide whether the rash is a photosensitive 'butterfly' rash that occurs in one-third of SLE patients or is due to erysipelas/facial cellulitis. Important information to elicit is whether this woman has ever had a similar rash or a change in cosmetic product, facial trauma, or increased sun exposure.

The history of a rapidly spreading facial demarcated rash in a systemically unwell patient with high C-reactive protein (CRP) should raise suspicion of facial erysipelas. Classically, CRP is relatively normal, and the erythrocyte sedimentation rate (ESR) is markedly raised in acute SLE flares, so a markedly raised CRP in this case suggests an active infection.

A rheumatology consultation should be sought. In some instances, complement level and anti–double-stranded DNA antibody titre are useful, as they correlate with SLE disease activity. In this scenario, blood cultures should be taken and antibiotics and fluid resuscitation should be instigated without any delay. Rapid improvement should be expected; otherwise, it is important to look out for intracranial complications such as cavernous sinus thrombosis and orbital cellulitis—known important complications of facial erysipelas.

 KEY POINTS

1. An acute SLE flare should be differentiated from other complications such as sepsis in an acutely unwell patient.
2. If aggressive SLE flares occur frequently and early in the disease course, mortality risk is high.

CASE 95: SELF-LIMITING GENERALISED SEIZURES

History

An unkempt man has been brought to the emergency department, having been found col-lapsed in the street. Earlier he was seen sitting in the street confused and agitated. An empty 2-litre cider bottle was found in his possession. He is unable to give a history.

Initial Treatment

Shortly after arrival the man started having a generalised seizure which self-terminated in 3 minutes. Supplemental oxygen was given, and intravenous access was established. His Glasgow Coma Scale score after the seizure was 4/15 (E1, V2, M1). While the attending doctor was assessing this man, he began to have another generalised seizure. A dose of lorazepam 4 mg was given intravenously and was repeated after 10 minutes as he continued to have seizures.

INVESTIGATIONS

- Arterial blood gas sample

	15 L oxygen	Normal range
pH	7.25	7.35–7.45
pO_2	25	9.3–13.3 kPa
pCO_2	3.2	4.7–6.0 kPa
Lactate	4.0	<2 mmol/L
HCO_3	19	22–26 mmol/L
Base excess	−8	−3 to +3 mmol/L

? QUESTION

1. What should be the immediate management plan for this patient?

DOI: 10.1201/9781003241171-95

ANSWER

The immediate management should consist of the following:

A: Maintain a patent airway by laying this man in the recovery position. If possible: chin lift, controlled suction, oropharyngeal airway if appropriate.

B: Apply high-flow oxygen and assess respiratory rate and targeted chest assessment.

C: Monitor heart rate and blood pressure, and fluid-resuscitate as appropriate.

D: Glucose is very important in any patient presenting with seizure and should be assessed immediately. Assess for focal neurological signs suggesting a focal brain lesion.

Any sick patient should be monitored in a high-dependency area. A useful acronym is MOVE:

M: Monitoring (cardiorespiratory)

O: give Oxygen

V: establish Venous access

E: perform 12-lead ECG

An arterial blood gas is always a useful test when a patient is unwell. The blood gas results of this patient show that he has an acidosis (pH <7.35). The patient is well oxygenated (on 15 L of O_2 via a non-rebreathing mask), and his pCO_2 is slightly lower than normal, so this is not a respiratory acidosis. His bicarbonate level is low, and his lactate level is high. This is a metabolic acidosis, which has probably resulted from earlier tissue hypoxia.

The National Institute for Health and Clinical Excellence pathway (treating prolonged or repeated seizures and status epilepticus) consists of a useful protocol for the management of acute seizure and status epilepticus. All practitioners of acute medicine should be familiar with the protocol.

Once a seizure is identified, always shout for help because it is impossible to execute ABCD + MOVE on your own. Look at your watch and note the time because it is useful in deciding what to do next.

Convulsive status epilepticus is defined as a seizure lasting more than 5 minutes or a patient having repeat seizures without regaining consciousness in between. Although the timeline on a conventional seizure treatment algorithm is very helpful, it is important to 'anticipate' rather than waiting for the next timepoint on the guideline to act (e.g. it takes time to draw up a lorazepam and phenytoin infusion). The timepoints serve as a guide only; in some circumstances it will be appropriate to expedite or delay a treatment according to the clinical situation. In this patient, intravenous dextrose and thiamine should be given, as there is a suspicion of alcohol-related seizure. Try to look for clues for seizure; for example, look for signs of head trauma (subdural or extradural haematoma), stroke, poisoning (methanol, ethylene glycol, paracetamol, etc.), or infection (encephalitis, meningitis). Correct hypotension and metabolic abnormalities as swiftly as possible.

Lorazepam is the preferred benzodiazepine in the United Kingdom as the first-line treatment of acute seizure. Lorazepam reaches a peak plasma concentration after 5 minutes, with peak central nervous system (CNS) effects by 30 minutes. Although intravenous diazepam is more rapid in onset of action, the significantly longer duration of action of lorazepam makes it a preferable drug, as it is effective for up to 5–8 hours. Diazepam has a shorter duration in the CNS, as it rapidly distributes in fat and tissues. Lorazepam should be given in a bolus at a maximum dose of 4 mg, and this can be repeated once in 10–20 minutes if seizures are not terminated. In instances where intravenous access is not possible, rectal diazepam 10 mg should be given. Peak concentration is reached in 10–20 minutes when diazepam is given rectally. If the seizure is terminated and the patient is able to swallow safely, they should be given their usual antiepileptic if they are known to have a diagnosis of epilepsy.

Intravenous phenytoin should be prepared as soon as possible when a repeated dose of benzodiazepine is given, as in the patient described. At this point the status epilepticus is established, and anaesthetists and the intensive care team should be alerted. Give phenytoin (15 mg/kg at a rate of 50 mg/min) as soon as it is feasible if the seizure is continuing. In refractory status epilepticus, a general anaesthetic drug such as thiopentone or propofol is often used. All agents used in the treatment of acute seizure have significant negative inotropic effects, so close cardiovascular monitoring is needed. Phenytoin is itself a class Ib Vaughan-Williams antiarrhythmic, and although its use in arrhythmia is obsolete, it acts on the cardiac sodium channel and shortens action potential; therefore ECG monitoring is needed. Cardiac patients especially with conduction abnormalities should be given phenytoin with caution. Phenytoin should be given into a large vein if possible, as it is very alkaline and may cause phlebitis: this can be quite severe and cause a 'purple glove syndrome'. Phenytoin should be diluted with normal saline, as dextrose solution causes precipitation. Blood sugar should be monitored regularly, as phenytoin can potentially cause both hyperglycaemia and hypoglycaemia.

When seizures are under control, consider neuroimaging to identify the underlying cause of presentation. All patients with a first seizure should receive follow-up and driving advice.

 KEY POINT

1. The treatment algorithm of generalised seizure and status epilepticus is important to learn, as it is a common medical emergency.

History

A 19-year-old man attends the emergency department with a 1-day history of rapid onset of multiple small itchy and painful skin rash and blisters on the hands and feet. This is associated with sore throat, mouth, and lips and red eyes. He also complains of malaise which started 3–4 days before the onset of the skin lesions. He is fit, with no previous history of any skin disorder or allergy. Seven days earlier he twisted his ankle while playing football and had taken paracetamol and ibuprofen for a few days.

Examination

This young man looks unwell. He has conjunctival injection bilaterally. There are multiple irregular erosions in the mouth and on the lips that are tender with haemorrhagic crusting. There are multiple, 1-cm-diameter, target-like lesions on the hands and feet. Nikolsky's sign is positive over the same distribution. The rest of the cardiorespiratory, abdominal, and neurological examinations were unremarkable. There was no lymphadenopathy. Observations: temperature 37.9°C, heart rate 120 beats/min, blood pressure 80/50 mmHg, respiratory rate 24/min, SpO$_2$ 99% on room air.

INVESTIGATIONS

White cells	16.0
Haemoglobin	13.2
Platelets	262
Sodium	135
Potassium	3.5
Urea	6.2
Creatinine	72
C-reactive protein	112

? QUESTIONS

1. What is the diagnosis?
2. How would you manage this young man?

ANSWERS

The skin lesions are typical of erythema multiforme (EM), which are painful and itchy target-like lesions that are each less than 1 cm diameter in size. EM with conjunctivitis and mucosal ulcers (in this case, mouth ulcers) are characteristic of Stevens-Johnson syndrome (SJS) and toxic epidermal necrolysis (TEN). SJS and TEN have similar pathophysiological processes and clinically differ on the extent of dermatological and mucosal involvement. The extent of skin lesion in SJS is usually less than 10% of the body surface area (BSA). TEN is a severe form of SJS where over 30% BSA is affected. Overlapping SJS/TEN is defined as 10%–30% BSA affected. SJS/TEN can be caused by infection (e.g. herpes virus, human immunodeficiency virus, *Mycoplasma pneumoniae* and group A streptococcus), lymphoma, or drugs (e.g. antibiotics, anticonvulsants, non-steroidal anti-inflammatory drug, and allopurinol). The lag time between drug exposure and symptoms can vary between 7 and 21 days. The dermis separates from the epidermis in SJS/TENS, causing extensive erosion and blisters (positive Nikolsky's sign). The oral, conjunctival, respiratory, gastrointestinal, and urogenital mucosae can also be involved, leading to lip adhesion, corneal erosions, laryngeal oedema and erosions, respiratory failure, gastrointestinal bleeding, urinary retention, sepsis, and multi-organ failure. Scoring systems such as SCORTEN (SCORe of Toxic Epidermal Necrolysis) is helping in predicting the prognosis.

The first step in the management of this patient is to stop the culprit drug, which is likely to be the ibuprofen. Immediate dermatology, ophthalmology, and intensive care input are required. The condition typically progresses over several days, so close monitoring and regular re-evaluation are essential. Transfer to a specialised burns unit may be required in the most severe cases.

The patient should be treated in a temperature-controlled (25–28°C) humidified side room with specialised mattress. Regular dressings of the skin lesions with topical antibacterial agents is required to prevent superinfection. Nutritional support may be required in patients who have severe oral lesions. Proton pump inhibitors can minimise the risk of upper gastrointestinal bleeding. The eyes may need topical steroids and medical amniotic membrane cover to prevent visual impairment. This patient is tachycardic and hypotensive, and he needs prompt treatment with intravenous fluids. Empirical systemic antibiotics should be started if there is evidence of infection. High-dose corticosteroids, ciclosporin, and intravenous immunoglobulin are sometimes used, but there is no definitive evidence of clinical benefit.

SJS/TENS is a serious adverse drug reaction, and this should be reported via the yellow card system online at the Medicines and Healthcare Products Regulatory Agency (MHRA) website.

🔑 **KEY POINTS**

- The presence of target-like lesions in the context of a drug reaction is highly suggestive of EM.
- SJS and TEN are dermatological emergencies that need to be treated promptly.
- Withdraw all implicated drug therapy as soon as possible.

CASE 97: SEIZURE

History

A 62-year-old woman presented with inferior ST-elevation myocardial infarction (STEMI). She was thrombolysed with tenecteplase, and she remained well for 72 hours. On the fourth day after admission she had a grand mal seizure that self-terminated in 3 minutes. After the fit she remained drowsy. She is known to have ischaemic heart disease and hypertension. Her current medications are aspirin 75 mg once daily; ramipril 2.5 mg once daily; bisoprolol 5 mg once daily; atorvastatin 40 mg once daily; GTN spray prn.

Examination

On examination it appears that she is snoring; however, her cardiorespiratory examination is otherwise normal. Her Glasgow Coma Scale (GCS) score is 6/15 (E2, V1, M3). Pupils are equal and reactive to light bilaterally and there are spontaneous eye movements. There is no neck stiffness. The tone in all limbs is slightly raised. Reflexes are reduced globally. Bilateral clonus is present, and both plantar responses are extensor. Observations: temperature 37.2°C, heart rate 120 beats/min, blood pressure 150/90 mmHg, respiratory rate 28/min, SaO_2 92% on room air.

🔍 INVESTIGATIONS

Arterial blood gas on room air:		Normal range
pH	7.36	7.35–7.45
pO_2	8.2	9.3–13.3 kPa
pCO_2	5.2	4.7–6.0 kPa
Lactate	2.0	<2 mmol/L
HCO_3	23	22–26 mmol/L
Base excess	−2	−3 to +3 mmol/L

❓ QUESTIONS

1. What is the immediate concern with this patient?
2. How would you further investigate this woman's current problem?

DOI: 10.1201/9781003241171-97

ANSWERS

This woman had a recent myocardial infarction (MI), which, unusually, was treated with thrombolytics. First-line treatment for STEMI should always aim to be primary percutaneous coronary intervention (PCI) unless there are clear reasons for opting for thrombolysis, such as no access to a primary PCI centre. The patient had a self-terminating seizure, and her consciousness level was depressed. An immediate concern is her snoring, which is indicative of partial upper airway obstruction. She should have an airway adjunct (e.g. oropharyngeal airway) inserted immediately and supplemental high-flow oxygen applied to bring up her oxygen saturation. She should be nursed in the recovery position for now.

It is important to check her blood sugar, as it is a rapidly reversible cause of a seizure. More importantly, reassess airway, breathing, and circulation until the patient is stabilised. She should be moved to a high-dependency area in the ward so that close monitoring is possible. Venous access should be established and blood taken to look for reversible causes of seizure such as electrolyte disturbances. Always perform a 12-lead ECG when feasible because 'seizure-like' activity (especially unwitnessed) could be caused by underlying cardiac arrhythmia (e.g. prolonged QT-interval syndrome could present as a morning tonic-clonic seizure). In addition, seizures can trigger cardiac arrhythmias.

Given the history of cardiovascular disease with target-organ damage (recent MI) and use of thrombolysis, the most important diagnosis to exclude here is a stroke. The presence of cardiovascular disease increases the probability of cerebrovascular pathology, or the mechanism might be a bleed related to the thrombolysis or embolus from thrombus in the left ventricle over an infarcted area. The incidence of stroke after thrombolysis is around 1%–1.5%, and most strokes occur within 5 days of the MI, with most cases of haemorrhage within 24 hours of MI and thrombolysis. The given collection of neurological signs is not 'classical' for a stroke, and it is not possible to determine which circulation (anterior versus posterior arterial territories) is affected. However, most of the findings could be explained by a recent seizure. Findings of decorticate response (flexor response) to external stimuli and seizure in the context of a stroke suggest a large lesion above the brainstem. With this level of GCS score and impending airway obstruction, an urgent anaesthetic assessment should be sought with a view to intubation.

Once she is stable, she should have urgent neuroimaging (CT or MRI) to look for evidence of intracerebral haemorrhage. The key to management of any post-stroke patient is attention to:

- Reversal of vascular risk factors—anticoagulation for atrial fibrillation and antiplatelet therapy after ischaemic stroke, good blood pressure control, cholesterol and glucose control, internal carotid endarterectomy if indicated
- Nutritional support
- Focused neurorehabilitation from a stroke unit with multi-disciplinary support—swallowing assessment, pressure sore prevention, temperature monitoring, deep vein thrombosis prophylaxis, speech and language therapy, physiotherapy and occupational therapy

In cases of intracerebral haemorrhage, anticoagulants and antiplatelets are contraindicated, and they should be withheld. Start insulin for hyperglycaemia to main blood sugar concentration between 4 and 11 mmol/L. Rapid blood pressure lowering is recommended to a target of systolic blood pressure 130–140 mmHg unless there is a clear contraindication (e.g. underlying structural brain disorder such as tumour or aneurysm, GCS <6, planned imminent neurosurgery to evacuate haematoma, and those who have a poor expected prognosis). Neurosurgery has little role except in selected cases and in those who develop hydrocephalus.

Some patients who present with an acute ischaemic stroke are eligible for thrombolysis; however, there is a strict national guideline to adhere to (standardised inclusion/exclusion criteria, the use of National Institutes of Health stroke scale assessment prior to thrombolysis). Alteplase, a tissue plasminogen activator, is used in the United Kingdom. In some circumstances it can be used up to 4.5 hours from the onset of symptoms and signs. Intense monitoring during and after thrombolysis is necessary, including blood pressure monitoring to look out for signs of cerebral haemorrhage and anaphylaxis—known complications associated with thrombolysis. More recently, in more selected cases endovascular treatment with mechanical thrombectomy to remove the thrombus is available in selected centres.

🔑 KEY POINTS

1. Stroke is a common medical emergency that carries high morbidity and mortality.
2. The field of stroke management is rapidly evolving. It is important to be aware of the different types of stroke syndromes and their treatment algorithms.

CASE 98: LOSS OF PAIN SENSATION

History

A 35-year-old man has presented with a severe burn to his right hand. He tipped some boiling water on to the hand a few hours earlier, which led to severe erythema and blisters, but he does not complain of any pain from the injury. Over the last month he has experienced mild shoulder pain, exacerbated by coughing, and bilateral leg stiffness resulting in walking difficulty. He works as a librarian. He has no medical, drug, travel, or smoking histories. He drinks fewer than 10 units of alcohol per week.

Examination

Cardiorespiratory and abdominal examinations are unremarkable. There is no rash or lymphadenopathy. Cranial nerve examination is normal, and no spinal tenderness is elicited. In the upper limb, tone is normal. His hands appear to have slight wasting bilaterally, with mild weakness, but other myotomes are within normal limits. There is no wrist tenderness. Reflexes in the arms are absent. Light touch sensation is intact throughout the upper limbs, but pain sensation is absent bilaterally from C4 to T4. In the lower limbs, the tone is elevated with ankle clonus bilaterally. Power is globally reduced to 4/5 (Medical Research Council scale), and there is hyperreflexia. All sensation modalities are intact in the lower limbs. Coordination and vibration sense are preserved in all limbs. Anal tone and perineal sensation are intact. A chest x-ray shows no abnormalities. Observations: temperature 36.5°C, heart rate 80 beats/min, blood pressure 105/70 mmHg, SaO_2 100% on room air.

🔍 INVESTIGATIONS

		Normal range
White cells	6.0	$4-11 \times 10^9$/L
Neutrophils	2.8	$2-7 \times 10^9$/L
Haemoglobin	13.0	13–18 g/dL
Platelets	250	$150-400 \times 10^9$/L
Sodium	137	135–145 mmol/L
Potassium	4.5	3.5–5.0 mmol/L
Urea	4.6	3.0–7.0 mmol/L
Creatinine	73	60–110 µmol/L
C-reactive protein	300	<5 mg/L
Bilirubin	20	5–25 µmol/L
Alanine transaminase	35	8–55 IU/L
Alkaline phosphatase	180	42–98 IU/L
Albumin	35	35–50 g/L
Creatine kinase	88	60–320 IU/L
Erythrocyte sedimentation rate	<10	Males, age/2; females, [age+10]/2
Antinuclear antibodies	Negative	
Antinuclear cytoplasmic antibodies	Negative	

❓ QUESTIONS

1. What is the differential diagnosis?
2. What should be the management plan?

DOI: 10.1201/9781003241171-98

ANSWERS

In approaching a neurological case, it is important to try to localise where the lesion(s) are within the neurological system. When investigating weakness, it can be divided into:

- Myopathy (i.e. not a neurological disorder)
- Neuromuscular junction disorder
- Peripheral nerve
- Radiculopathy/spinal cord lesion/myelopathy
- Lesion in the brainstem and/or cerebellum
- Cortical lesion

The patterns of presentation differ, and this helps to localise the lesion.

This patient's neurological findings can be summarised as:

- Spastic paraparesis in the lower limbs (as demonstrated by bilateral upper motor neuron signs)
- Dissociated sensory loss in the upper limbs (i.e. spinothalamic impairment but intact posterior column)
- Absent upper limb reflexes with hand muscle wasting

Putting all this together suggests the lesion is within the spinal cord at the level of the cervical and upper thoracic cord. This will produce a segmental effect, as demonstrated by lower motor neuron signs in the upper limbs and long-tract effect, as demonstrated by upper motor neuron signs below the level of the spinal cord lesion.

Having established the site of lesion within the neurological system, the next step is to find out what type of cord lesion this is. The common causes of cord lesions are tumours, infection, disc disease and spondylosis, haematoma, or cystic lesions. Except for disc disease and spondylosis, most of these pathological processes can occur in the extradural, intradural, or intramedullary space. All lesions within the spinal cord can produce local segmental damage and long-tract effects (i.e. damage/interruption to ascending and descending tracts within the cord).

With regard to local segmental damage, the lesions can affect (i) a nerve root (radiculopathy), which leads to severe, sharp, shooting, burning pain at that nerve root distribution and is aggravated by movement, straining, and coughing or (ii) cord (myelopathy), leading to a dull ache which is continuous, unaffected by movement, and may radiate into the whole leg or even one half of the body. Bone pathology tends to cause localised tenderness, which is reproducible by palpation of the affected area. Long-tract effects are dependent on which long tract is affected (spinothalamic, posterior column, spinocerebellar, or corticospinal tracts). In addition, damage to the sympathetic outflow at the level of T1 or the cervical cord may lead to Horner's syndrome. Bladder symptoms occur when both sides of the spinal cord are affected; usually they start with difficulty in initiating micturition before retention symptoms develop.

The combinations of presenting symptoms are also reflective of segmental damage within the affected cord. Cord lesion can be divided into (i) extrinsic compressive lesions, (ii) central cord lesions, and (iii) cauda equina lesions. For extrinsic compressive lesions, the long-tract effects depend on the location of the tumour. For example, a posterior tumour causes ipsilateral posterior column lesions first (light touch, proprioception, and vibration sensory loss), and, as it expands, it may cause further direct pressure effects or ischaemia to the neighbouring tracts—so it may cause ipsilateral corticospinal tract lesions (upper motor neuron signs) and then contralateral spinothalamic tract lesions (pain and temperature loss). If half of the spinal cord is affected, then it produces a combination of symptoms consistent with Brown-Séquard syndrome.

In contrast to extrinsic compressive lesions, the central cord lesions produce a different set of long-tract signs. The centrality of the lesion means that the medially situated fibres are involved first. As the spinothalamic tract decussates at the level of the spinal cord, central cord lesions cause bilateral sensory loss at the level of the lesion initially. With a cervical central cord lesion, the pattern of spinothalamic damage may expand to a 'cape' or 'suspended' pattern (with pain and temperature sensory deficit spared in the sacral distribution even with large central lesion) due to the peripheral location of sacral fibres within the spinothalamic tract. As the central cord lesion expands, corticospinal tracts are involved, leading to lower motor neuron lesions at the level of the spinal cord affected (e.g. hand muscle wasting) and upper motor neuron signs below the level of lesions (e.g. spastic paraparesis). Posterior column signs appear late.

Cauda equina lesions typically affect the lumbosacral areas. If lesions are affecting the sacral nerve roots, they cause saddle anaesthesia and bladder symptoms earlier than other lesions.

This man's symptoms and signs are consistent with a central spinal cord lesion. The combination of dissociated sensory loss and spastic paraparesis is highly suggestive of a cystic lesion known as syringomyelia. Other differential diagnoses are cystic intramedullary tumours, infection, and haematoma. Subacute combined degeneration of the cord and multiple sclerosis can sometimes produce a similar collection of symptoms.

Syringomyelia is a rare disorder with a prevalence of 8.4 cases per 100,000 population. An abnormal cerebrospinal fluid (CSF)–filled cavity known as a syrinx develops in the spinal cord. If a syrinx develops within the brainstem, the condition is termed syringobulbia. Syringomyelia is associated with Arnold-Chiari malformation, which is a developmental abnormality of the brainstem and cerebellum: the cerebellar tonsils herniate through the foramen magnum. The pathophysiology of syringomyelia is incompletely understood.

Magnetic resonance imaging of the brain and spinal cord is the investigation of choice (Figure 98.1), which will demonstrate the characteristic syrinx, the extent of the lesion, and rule out other conditions as mentioned earlier. CSF sampling is relatively contraindicated owing to the risk of herniation. The natural history of this condition is variable, and neurosurgery is considered but is not curative because, despite best effort, at least 33% of patients suffer progressive deterioration.

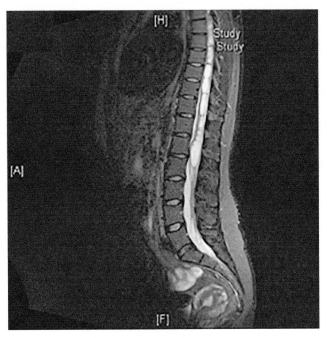

Figure 98.1

🔑 **KEY POINTS**

1. It is important to recognise the different patterns of neurological presentation in order to make an accurate neurological diagnosis.
2. Syrinx cavities can often be managed conservatively.
3. The extent of the lesion does not necessarily associate with the severity of the effects on neurological signs or symptoms.

CASE 99: SHORTNESS OF BREATH IN A RETURNING TRAVELLER

History

A 65-year-old man has presented to the emergency department with a 1-day history of generalised headache, shortness of breath, fever, rigours, productive cough, right-sided pleuritic chest pain, myalgia, and watery diarrhoea. He returned from Kuala Lumpur 3 days ago after a 5-day holiday with his family. He stayed in the city and did not visit the countryside. His hotel was air-conditioned, and he ate cooked meals there. His wife, who was travelling with him, also presented with a similar illness. He is normally fit and well with no past medical history.

Examination

The man is visibly tachypnoeic and appears disorientated in time and place. There is no rash or signs of meningeal irritation. He feels hot to the touch, and his pulse is fast and regular but bounding in character. On auscultation of his chest there is bronchial breathing and coarse crackles in the right mid and lower zones posteriorly. The rest of the cardiorespiratory, abdominal, and neurological examinations are unremarkable. A chest x-ray is shown in Figure 99.1. Observations: temperature 40°C, heart rate 130 beats/min, blood pressure 108/55 mmHg, respiratory rate 32/min, SaO_2 90% on room air.

🔍 INVESTIGATIONS

		Normal range
White cells	20.0	$4-11 \times 10^9$/L
Neutrophils	18	$2-7 \times 10^9$/L
Haemoglobin	15.0	13–18 g/dL
Platelets	188	$150-400 \times 10^9$/L
Sodium	129	135–145 mmol/L
Potassium	3.9	3.5–5.0 mmol/L
Urea	15	3.0–7.0 mmol/L
Creatinine	155	60–110 µmol/L
C-reactive protein	300	<5 mg/L
Bilirubin	20	5–25 µmol/L
Alanine aminotransferase	35	8–55 IU/L
Alkaline phosphatase	180	42–98 IU/L
Albumin	35	35–50 g/L
Creatine kinase	568	60–320 IU/L
Arterial blood gas on room air:		
pH	7.48	7.35–7.45
pO_2	7.9	9.3–13.3 kPa
pCO_2	3.2	4.7–6.0 kPa
Lactate	4.0	<2 mmol/L
HCO_3	24	22–26 mmol/L
Base excess	−3	−3 to +3 mmol/L

DOI: 10.1201/9781003241171-99

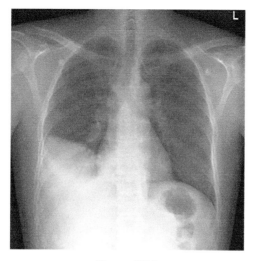

Figure 99.1

? | **QUESTIONS**

1. What is the diagnosis?
2. What should be the management plan?

ANSWERS

This man's clinical presentation and investigation results are highly suggestive of community-acquired pneumonia. He has bronchial breathing indicating consolidation. His chest x-ray shows opacification in the right lower zone. This obscures the diaphragm, but not the right heart border, indicating that it is likely to be in the right lower lobe. It contains an air bronchogram confirming consolidation.

CURB 65 is one of the most commonly used tools for assessment of community-acquired pneumonia severity. It is a useful adjunct, but should not replace thorough clinical assessment. CURB 65 stands for: C = confusion; U = Urea ≥7 mmol/L; R = Respiratory rate >30/min; B = Blood pressure systolic <90 or diastolic <60 mmHg; 65 = age ≥65 years. Mortality approaches 83% if all four CURB components are present. CURB 65 is also a useful tool to decide whether to manage a patient with pneumonia in the community or in a hospital environment. When the patient is managed in the community, appropriate patient and/or relative education and clinical review mechanisms should be in place.

The most important initial management plan is to ensure his hypoxia is corrected by high-flow oxygen as swiftly as possible. Intravenous fluids should also be prescribed. The patient should be monitored in a high-dependency area with continuous cardiorespiratory and urine output monitoring. The aim is to ensure oxygen saturation is >94% and respiratory rate <30/min. It is also important to monitor for clinical signs of respiratory depression secondary to exhaustion. Patients with persistent hypoxia, signs of exhaustion, or shock should be transferred to a critical care unit as soon as possible for intubation and intermittent positive pressure ventilation and circulatory support. In respiratory failure secondary to pneumonia, non-invasive mask/helmet continuous positive airway pressure devices are a useful adjunct while awaiting invasive ventilation, but this should not delay intubation.

Antibiotics should be given at the earliest opportunity and should be no later than 4 hours after presentation to hospital. As with all antibiotic prescriptions, it is essential to establish a history of antibiotic allergy. When taking an allergy history, it is important to establish the nature of the drug allergy. If the allergy history is unclear, it is important to avoid the class of drugs in the acute setting with a view to allergy testing to clarify the nature of the allergy when the patient has recovered. Microbiology investigations, including sputum and blood cultures, should be taken, although it should not delay the initiation of antibiotics. Performing sputum cultures whilst on antibiotic treatment is unlikely to be helpful. In all severe cases of pneumonia, urinary pneumococcal antigen, urinary *Legionella* antigen, and *Mycoplasma* serology/sputum polymerase chain reaction (PCR) assay should be considered. Concurrently, respiratory viral pathogens are routinely screened for using nasopharyngeal swabs and PCR-based 'respiratory viral panels'. This is especially relevant in all pneumonia cases to identify and treat SARS-CoV2 cases, both for early antiviral treatment initiation and isolation. Similarly, positive influenza cases are also treated with specific antiviral treatments.

This man has presented with classic symptoms of fever with evidence of extrapulmonary manifestations such as headache, myalgia, and watery diarrhoea. His blood test also reveals an elevated liver enzyme profile and acute kidney injury. While all these features could be consistent with severe pneumonia leading to multi-organ injury or failure, atypical pneumonia should be suspected. Atypical pneumonia is not a distinctive clinical syndrome. Most, if not all, atypical pneumonias present with classical pneumonic symptoms (fever, productive cough, and shortness of breath), so it is hard to differentiate clinically. Atypical pneumonia is a term used to describe pneumonia caused by (i) *Mycoplasma pneumoniae*, (ii) *Chlamydophila pneumoniae*, (iii) *Chlamydophila psittaci*, (iv) *Coxiella burnetii*, (v) *Legionella* spp., or (vi) *Francisella tularensi*. The term 'atypical pneumonia' remains useful to describe these pathogens, as their treatment and sometimes duration of antibiotic therapy are different from typical pathogens. Atypical pathogens are intracellular pathogens and lack a bacterial cell wall, so they are not susceptible to β-lactam–based antibiotics. Atypical pneumonias are normally treated with macrolides, quinolones, or tetracycline classes of antibiotics.

In this case it is reasonable to suspect Legionnaire's disease from the travel history and a similar illness suffered by his wife. *Legionella* spp. are a group of gram-negative rods that are obligate or facultative intracellular bacteria. Transmission is usually via contaminated aerosol inhalation. Around half the cases are travel-related, and most UK cases occur predominantly over August and October each year from a combination of environmental and human behaviour over summer months. *Legionella* spp. thrive in the warmer waters of summer, and over this period there is usually an increased use of cooling towers and air conditioning units so that transmission is more frequent. *Legionella* infection has two distinctive clinical patterns. It can cause a rapid progressive illness and is seen more frequently in critically ill patients. It can also cause a mild self-limiting illness termed 'Pontiac fever'. The more severe form of *Legionella* disease can often lead to gastrointestinal, cardiac, and central nervous system manifestations, although other atypical organisms such as *C. psittaci*, *C. burnetiid*, and *M. pneumoniae* have distinctive extrapulmonary manifestations too.

In all patients diagnosed with community-acquired pneumonia, follow-up chest radiograph 6 weeks after the initial illness should be considered if there are persisting symptoms or clinical signs or a high risk of underlying malignancy. It is also important to note that *Legionella* is a notifiable illness, and all cases should be reported as per the UK Health Security Agency and local Health Protection Unit policy.

 KEY POINTS

1. *Legionella* disease is a notifiable illness.
2. It should be suspected in cases of severe community-acquired pneumonia.

CASE 100: A WOMAN "OFF HER LEGS"

History

An 82-year-old woman has been referred by her general practitioner (GP) for confusion and being "off her legs". She appears vacant and is unable to say why and how she came to the hospital. The referral letter states that she lives alone and has no immediate family. She was previously independent and walked with the aid of two sticks. Her medical history includes hypertension and osteoporosis. She is taking amlodipine 10 mg once daily and risedronate 35 mg once per week.

Examination

This elderly woman appears thin but healthy and well hydrated. There is a recent moderate-sized cut above her left eye, and there are several cuts and bruising on her arms and shins. She is unable to perform the 'get up and go' test, as she is unable to stand up. She is orientated in person only and is easily distracted by the surroundings, making physical examination very difficult. Her cardiovascular, respiratory, and abdominal examinations are unremarkable. There is no evidence of neck stiffness or photophobia. Her pupils are equal and dilated, and there are no abnormalities on examination of her cranial nerves. In her peripheral nervous system there is normal tone but globally depressed power (4/5). Reflexes are difficult to elicit, and she is unable to carry out clinical tests for coordination. Plantars are both withdrawn. Fundoscopy is within normal limits. A chest x-ray shows no abnormal features. Observations: temperature 36.8°C, heart rate 80 beats/min, blood pressure 138/65 mmHg, SaO_2 97% on room air.

INVESTIGATIONS

		Normal range
White cells	8.0	4–11 × 10⁹/L
Haemoglobin	12.8	13–18 g/dL
Platelets	250	150–400 × 10⁹/L
Sodium	125	135–145 mmol/L
Potassium	3.7	3.5–5.0 mmol/L
Urea	14.5	3.0–7.0 mmol/L
Creatinine	76	60–110 µmol/L
C-reactive protein	<5	<5 mg/L
Corrected calcium	2.2	2.2–2.6 mmol/L
Urine sodium	21 mmol/L	
Urine dipstick	1+ protein	

QUESTIONS

1. How would you interpret the low serum sodium?
2. What are the possible differential diagnoses for this woman's presentation?

DOI: 10.1201/9781003241171-100

ANSWERS

The low serum sodium interpreted with continued urinary sodium excretion is highly suggestive of the syndrome of inappropriate antidiuretic hormone secretion (SIADH). To make the diagnosis, it is necessary to ensure this patient is clinically euvolaemic without any other precipitants of hyponatraemia, such as diarrhoea and vomiting or diuretic use. The causes of SIADH are wide and can be classified into:

- Increased hypothalamic ADH production (cerebral trauma, infection, space-occupying lesion)
- Drugs—diuretics (which cause sodium depletion), chlorpropamide, carbamazepine, non-steroidal anti-inflammatories, tricyclic antidepressants, selective serotonin reuptake inhibitors (SSRIs), typical antipsychotics, monoamine oxidase inhibitors, chemotherapeutic agents
- Pulmonary diseases (carcinoma, pneumonia)
- Exogenous administration of ADH
- Idiopathic

This woman presented with delirium, which is one of the geriatric giants. Her 'get up and go' test may be difficult to interpret owing to her confusional state, but it would suggest a limited mobility and underlying risk of falling. Her physical signs of recent head trauma and bruising support a history of recent falls. Information from history, examination, and investigation results did not show any common precipitating causes of delirium, such as infection, intoxications, or metabolic derangements. Intracranial pathologies such as post-ictal state or space-occupying lesion may possibly explain her current presentation. Her clinical neurological signs are difficult to interpret: global weakness could be related to hyponatraemia, and confusion often makes eliciting neurological signs difficult.

As part of the workup for her delirium, it may be useful to obtain neuroimaging such as a CT brain to look for evidence of a space-occupying lesion, such as subdural haematoma or gliomas. If this test is negative, it may be worthwhile considering other tests such as EEG or lumbar puncture to exclude other intracranial causes of delirium. In this case a CT scan of the brain showed a right subdural haematoma (Figure 100.1). This can be managed conservatively or will require urgent neurosurgical intervention if there is reducing Glasgow Coma Scale (GCS) despite correction of hyponatraemia.

Collateral history is paramount to differentiate whether a presenting complaint of cognitive impairment is due to acute or chronic confusional state.

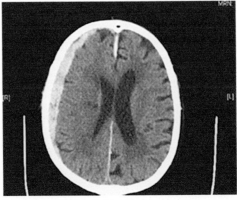

Figure 100.1 CT Head demonstrating a right subdural haematoma

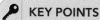 **KEY POINTS**

1. The diagnosis of SIADH should be made only after the patient's fluid status has been assessed.
2. A subdural haematoma can present insidiously in the elderly as delirium.

INDEX

A

ABC, *see* airway breathing circulation (ABC) pathway
ABCDE, *see* airway, breathing, circulation, disability, exposure
abdominal pain
  acute, 139
  alcohol binge, 265–266
  diarrhoea/fever, 250–252
  lower, 181–182
  malaise, 267–268
  recurrent, 75–76
  vomiting, 63–64
acidosis, 50
acute kidney injury (AKI), 140, 141, 207–209, 218, 254
  approach, 208–209
  creatinine (Cr), 208
  urine output (UO), 208
acute optic neuritis, treatment of, 260
acute respiratory distress syndrome (ARDS), 156
acute severe asthma attack, 214
acute tubular necrosis (ATN), 208
adrenocorticotropic hormone (ACTH), 218
adverse drug reaction, 5–7
airway, breathing, circulation, disability, exposure (ABCDE), 144, 148
airway breathing circulation (ABC) pathway, 6, 234
alcohol binge, abdominal pain, 265–266
alcohol dehydrogenase enzyme, 36
alcoholic liver disease, 120
alkaline phosphatase (ALP), 188
allergic bronchopulmonary aspergillosis (ABPA), 214
allopurinol, 166
  hypertension, 164
  Mycoplasma pneumoniae, 286
  xanthine oxidase inhibitor, 178
alopecia, pruritic rash, 247–248
alpha-blockade, 152
Alport's syndrome, 170
aminoglycoside toxicity, 209
amiodarone/digoxin, 240
amoxicillin
  drowsiness, 143
  for presumed community-acquired pneumonia, 5
  throat/fever, 100
ampicillin, sore throat/fever, 100
amyloidosis, 76, 170

anaemia, 56, 126
analgesia, pain, 32
anaphylaxis, 289
  acute management of, 6
  to penicillin-based antibiotic, 6
  signs of, 289
angiotensin-converting enzyme inhibitors (ACEIs), 2, 30, 96, 104, 116, 132, 162, 245, 273
angiotensin receptor blockers (ARBs), 162, 273
ankle arthritis, 132
ankle swelling, 61
anorexia nervosa
  lady with fatigue, 159–160
  metabolic alkalosis, 160
  psychiatric diagnosis, 160
antiarrhythmic treatment, 240
anticardiolipin IgG, 39
anticholinergics, 234
anticoagulation, 112
anti-D immunoglobulin, 124
antidiuretic hormone (ADH), 2
antifreeze, deliberate self-harm, 35–36
anti-glomerular basement membrane disease (anti-GBM), 162, 174
anti-helminth medication, 14
anti-IgE monoclonal antibodies, 128
anti-IL5 antibodies, 128
anti-inflammatory drug, non-steroidal, 286
antimitochondrial antibodies (AMA), 184, 188
anti-neutrophil cytoplasmic antibody (ANCA), 174
antinuclear antibodies (ANAs), 112, 162, 174, 184, 188
antinuclear cytoplasmic antibodies (ANCAs), 162
anti-smooth muscle antibodies (SMAs), 184, 188
antistreptococcal antibody titres (ASOTs), 100
a-1-antitrypsin deficiency (A1AD), 224
anti-tuberculous antibiotics, 184
anti–voltage gated calcium channel (VGCC), 130
anxiety, 147–149
aortic regurgitation, 72, 220
aortic stenosis, 104
apparent adverse drug reaction, 5–7
Arnold-Chiari malformation, 293